THIS BASEBALL JOURNAL BELONGS TO:

_____

DEDICATION

This Baseball Playbook is dedicated to all the Baseball Lovers out there who love to plan out their games, and document their findings in the process.

You are my inspiration for producing books and I'm honored to be a part of keeping all of your game day information and records organized.

How to use this Baseball Season Play Book:

This useful baseball season log book is a must-have for anyone that needs to record skill sets, games and memories! You will love this easy to use journal to track and record all your baseball game playing activities.

Each interior page includes space to record & track the following:

1. Date - Write down the date of practice or game day.
2. Coach's Focus - Use this space to fill in the coach's focus this week.
3. My Focus - Record by writing out your goal and focus this week.
4. Skill Set to Work On - Fill in the skills worked on this week.
5. Good Sportsmanship- Use the space provided to write down the ways you showed respect this week to coaches, players and parents.
6. Game Day Notes/Practice Notes- Stay on task by filling in who's at bat, inning pitched, or any important notes.

If you are new to the world of baseball playing or have been at it for a while, this baseball journal is a must have! Can make a great useful gift for anyone that loves to play baseball!

Have Fun!

PRE-SEASON PRACTICE

Date:

Location:

My focus this week is:

Coach's focus this week is:

Skills I need to work on this week are:

I showed good sportsmanship this week by:

How I feel starting out:

This week's practice notes:

PRACTICE DAY

Date:

Location:

My focus this week is:

Coach's focus this week is:

Skills I need to work on this week are:

I showed good sportsmanship this week by:

How I feel starting out:

This week's practice notes:

GAME DAY

Date:

Opponent:

Location:

My focus today is:

Coach's focus today is:

Skills I need to work on this week are:

I showed good sportsmanship today by:

How I feel starting out:

Game Day notes:

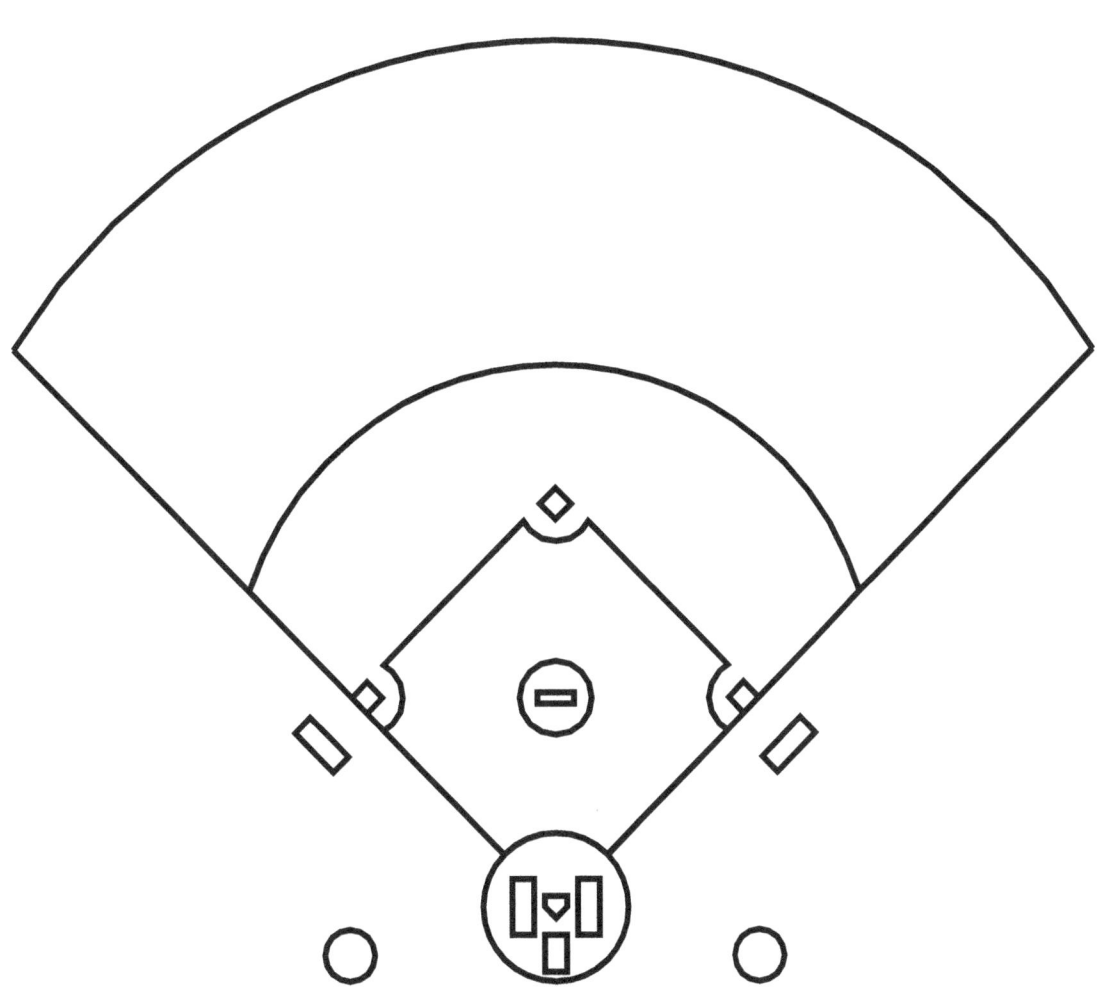

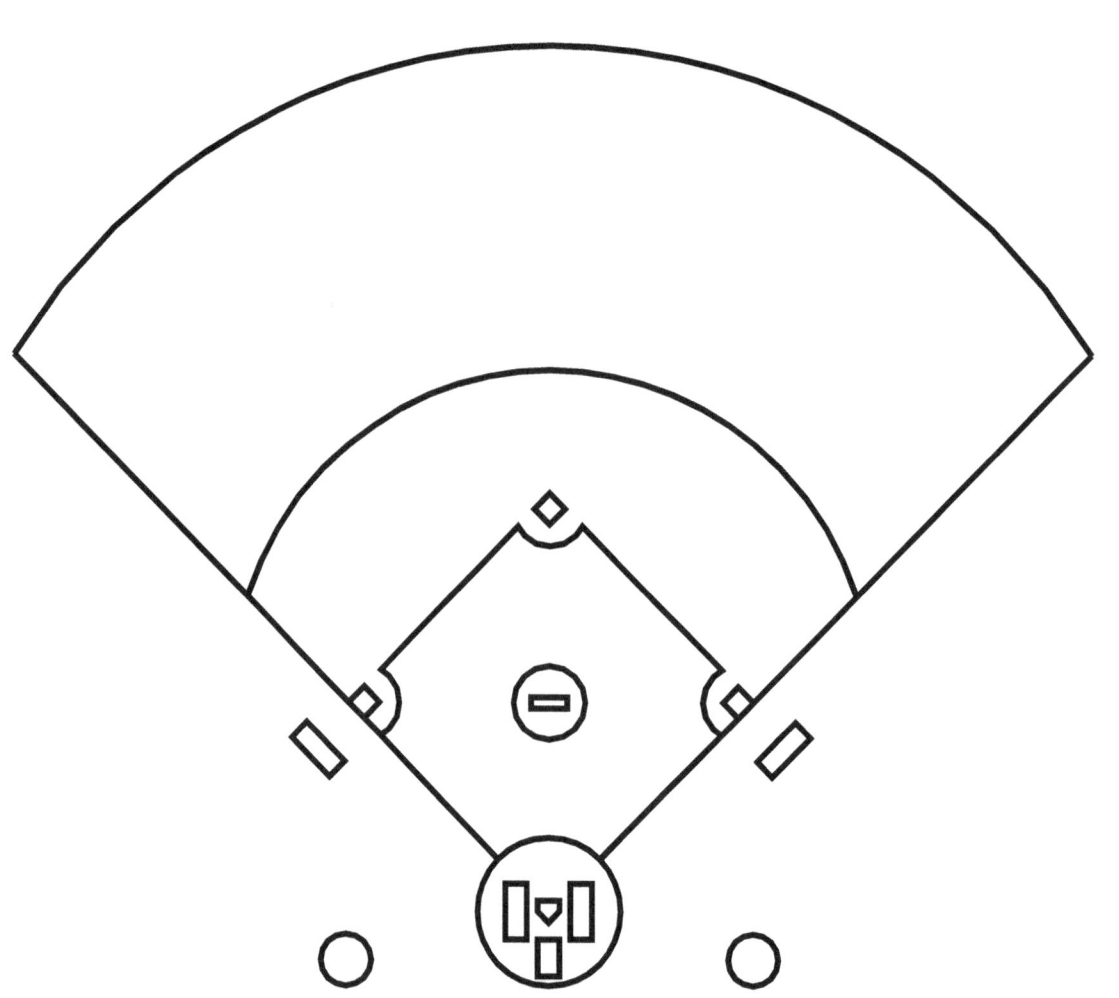

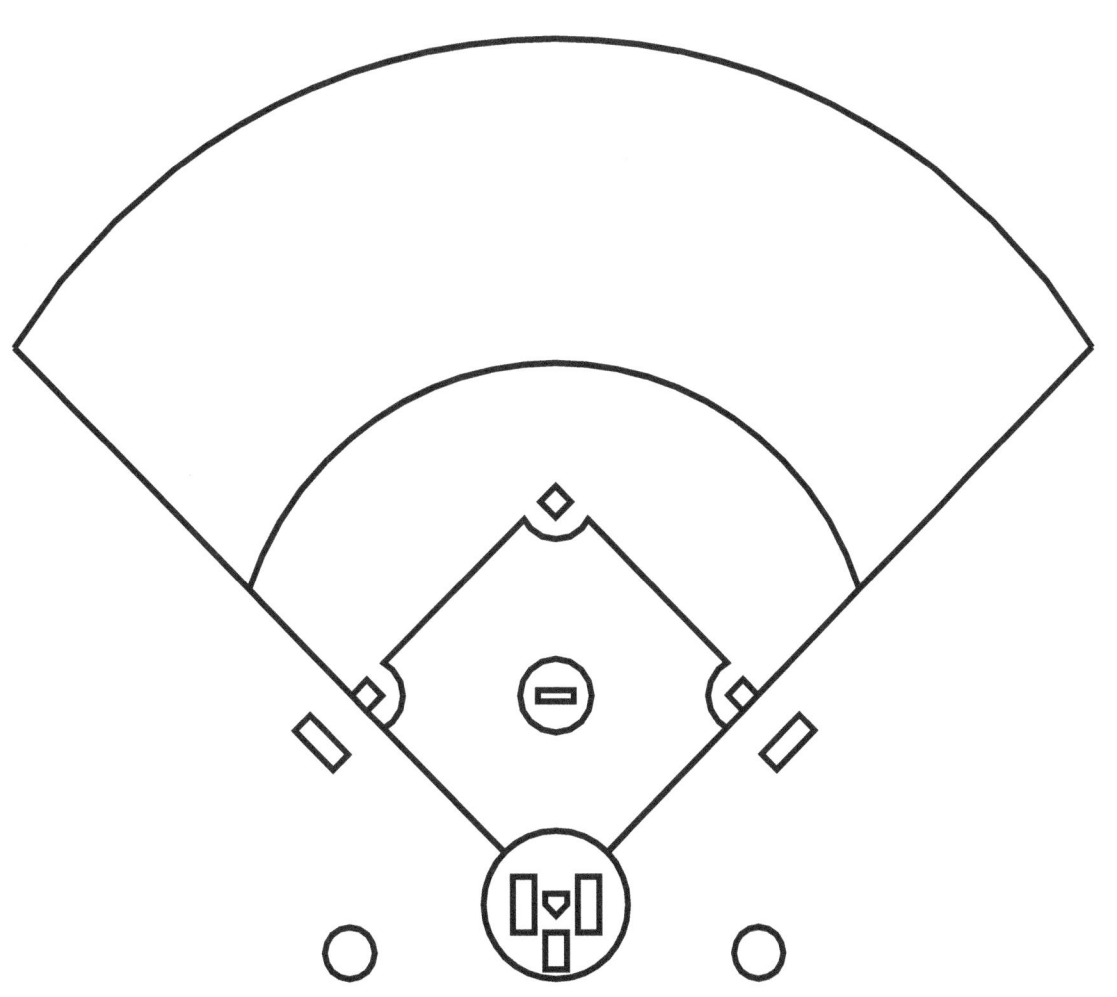

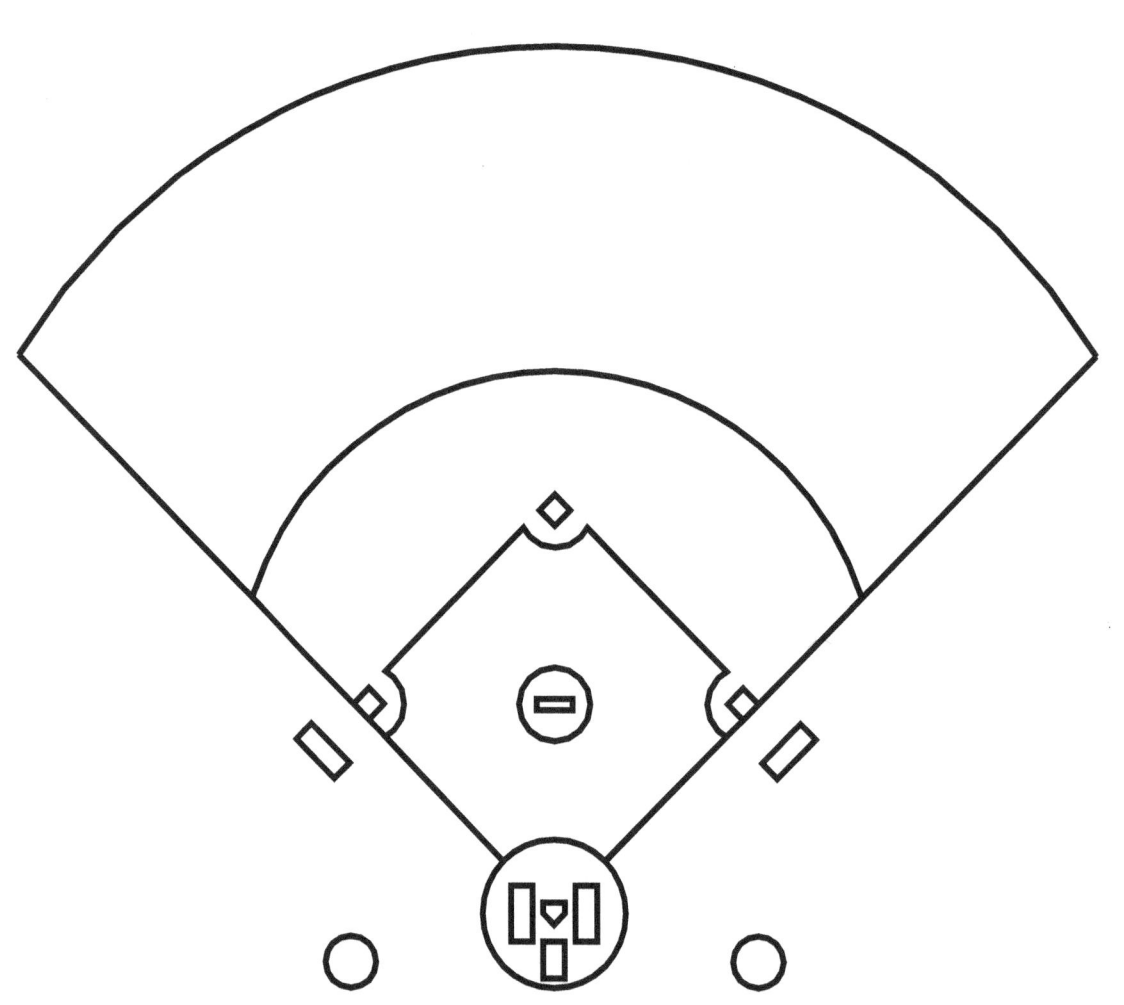

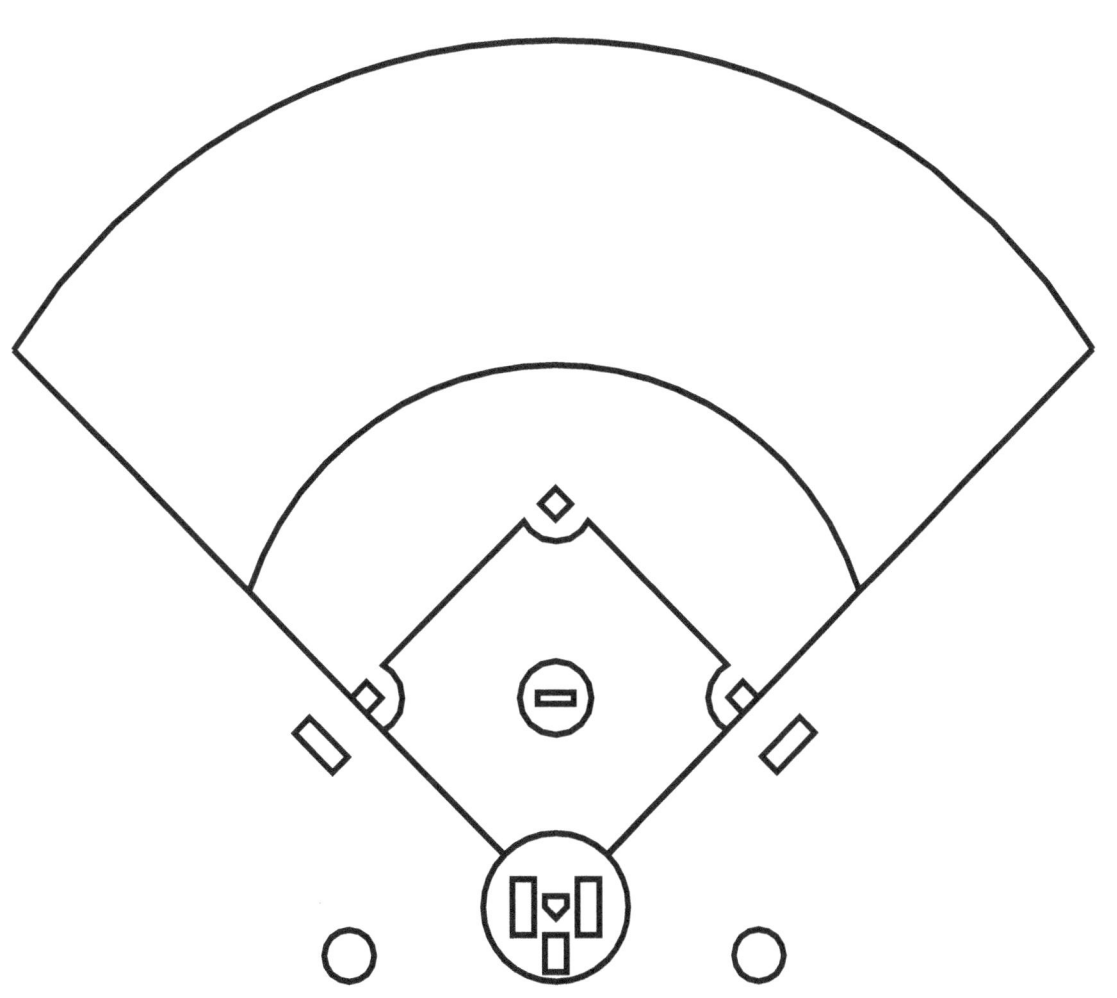

PRE-SEASON PRACTICE

Date:

Location:

My focus this week is:

Coach's focus this week is:

Skills I need to work on this week are:

I showed good sportsmanship this week by:

How I feel starting out:

This week's practice notes:

PRACTICE DAY

Date:

Location:

My focus this week is:

Coach's focus this week is:

Skills I need to work on this week are:

I showed good sportsmanship this week by:

How I feel starting out:

This week's practice notes:

GAME DAY

Date:

Opponent:

Location:

My focus today is:

Coach's focus today is:

Skills I need to work on this week are:

I showed good sportsmanship today by:

How I feel starting out:

Game Day notes:

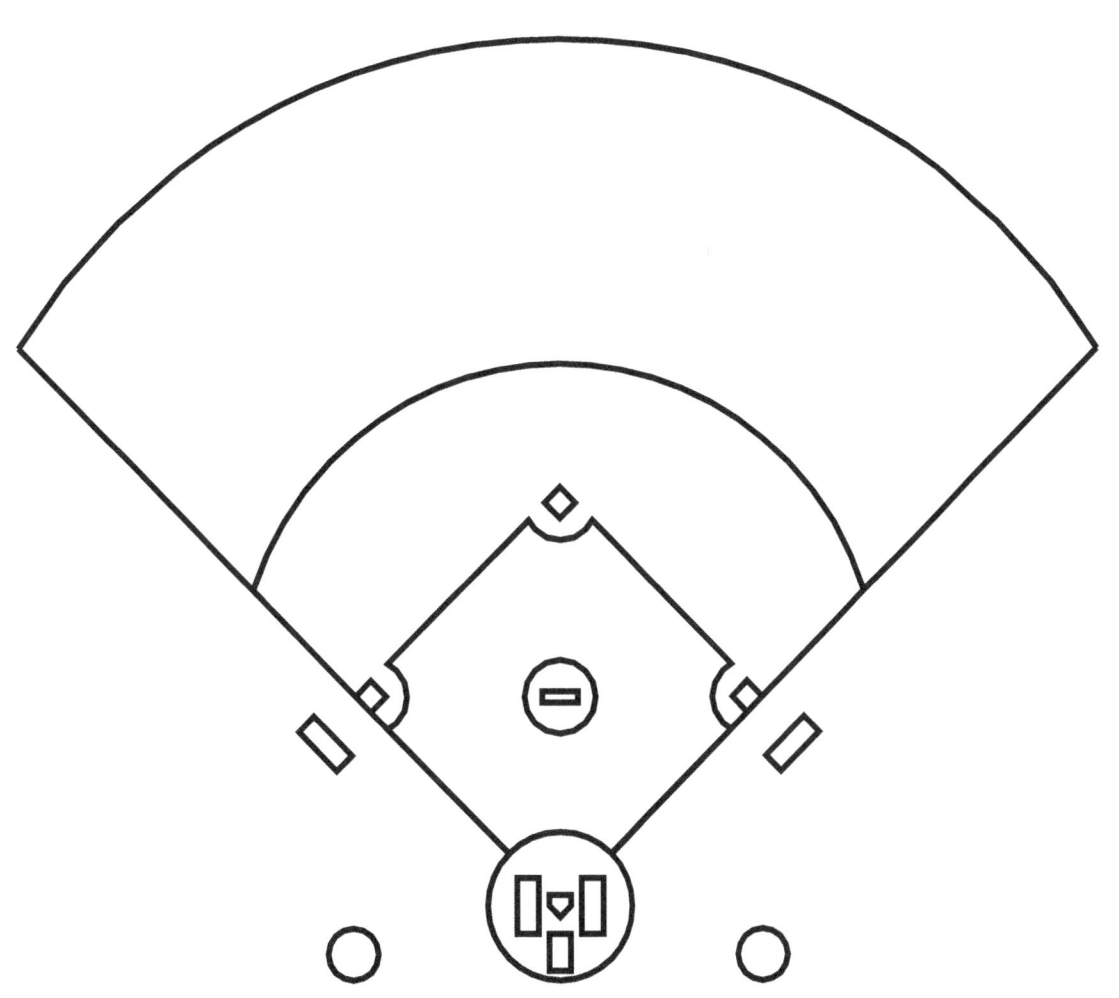

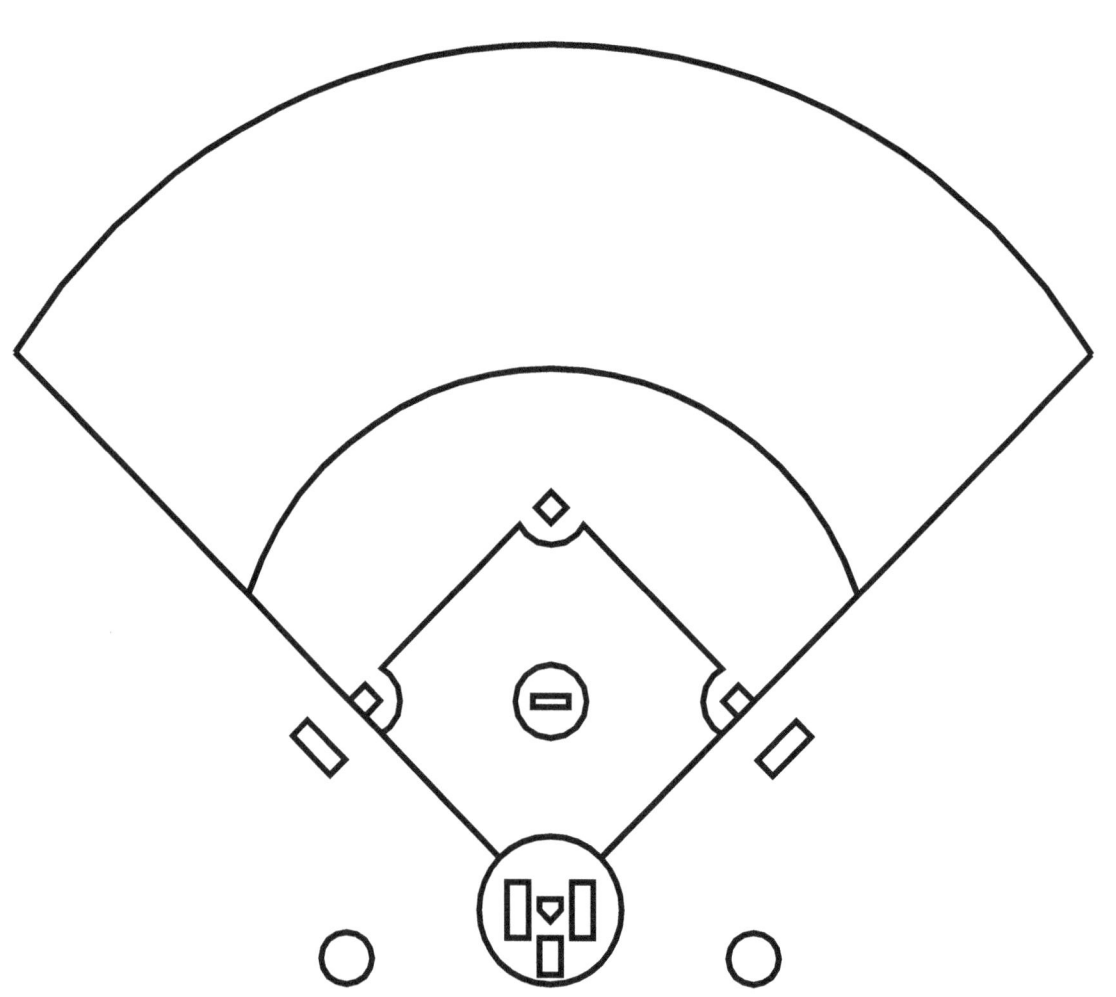

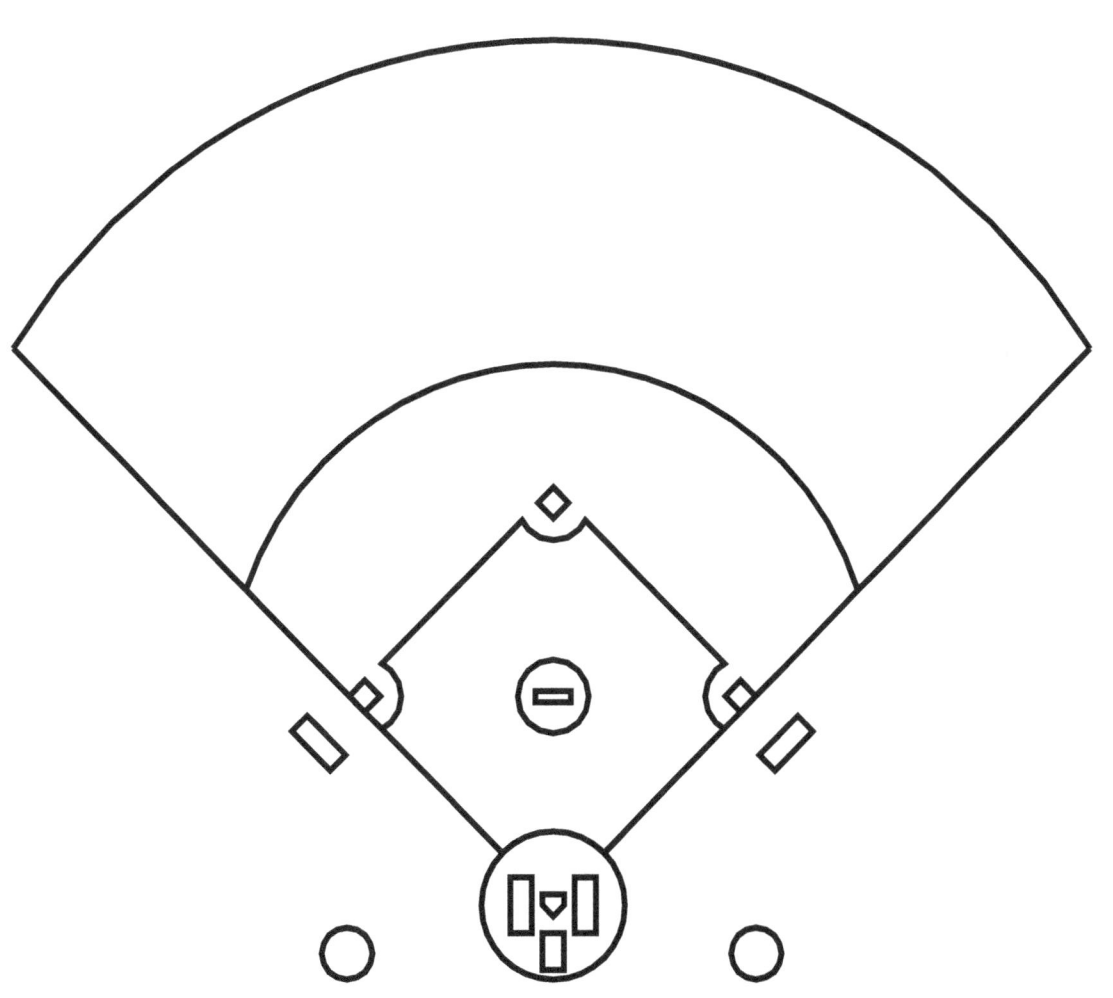

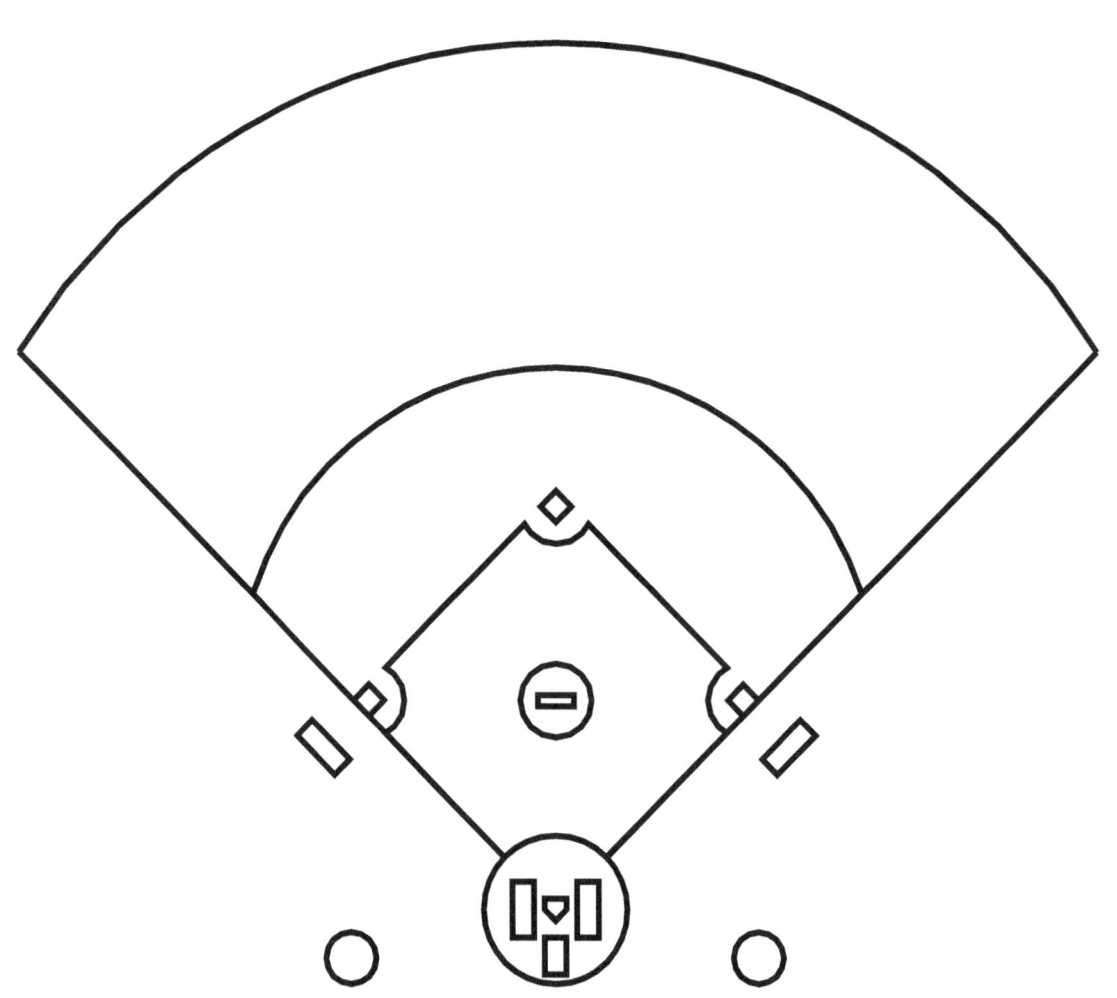

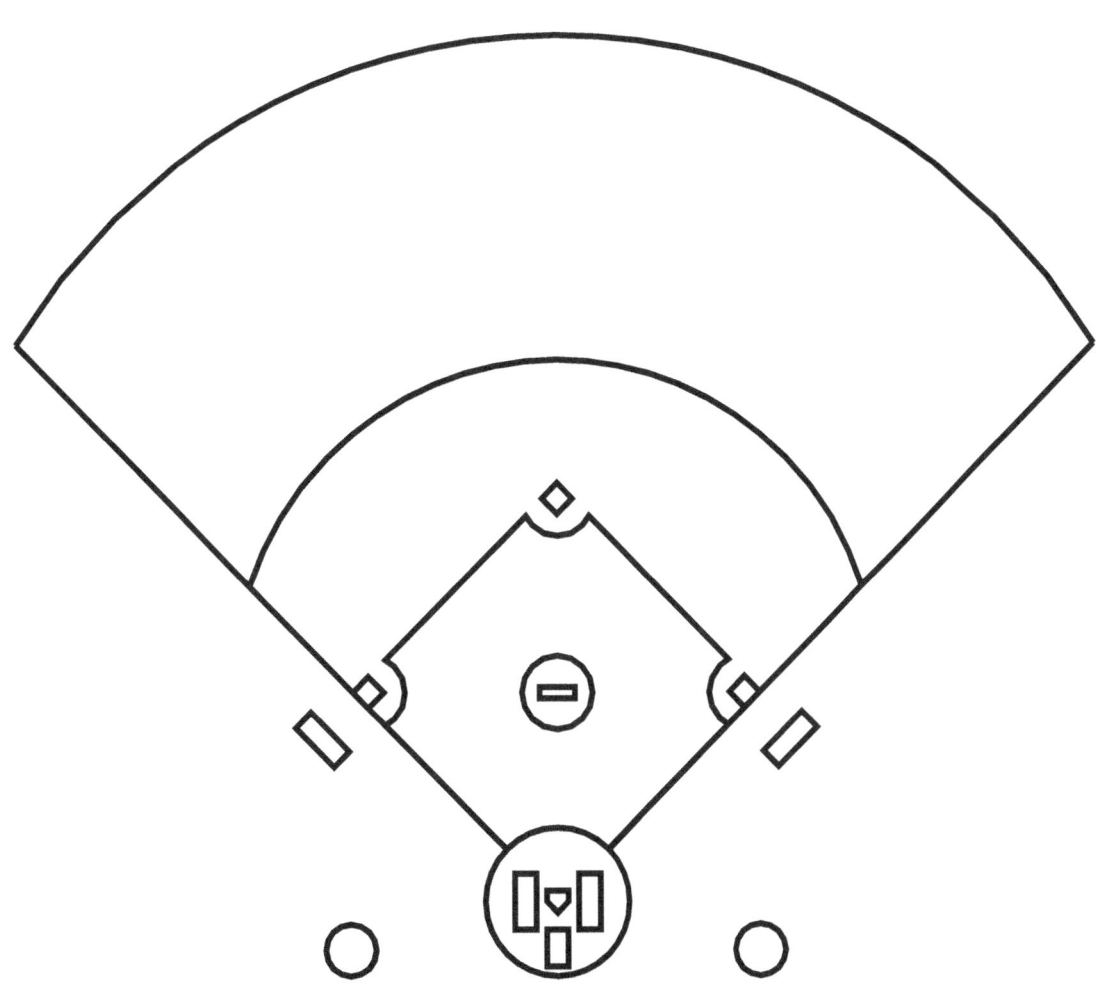

PRE-SEASON PRACTICE

Date:

Location:

My focus this week is:

Coach's focus this week is:

Skills I need to work on this week are:

I showed good sportsmanship this week by:

How I feel starting out:

This week's practice notes:

PRACTICE DAY

Date:

Location:

My focus this week is:

Coach's focus this week is:

Skills I need to work on this week are:

I showed good sportsmanship this week by:

How I feel starting out:

This week's practice notes:

GAME DAY

Date:

Opponent:

Location:

My focus today is:

Coach's focus today is:

Skills I need to work on this week are:

I showed good sportsmanship today by:

How I feel starting out:

Game Day notes:

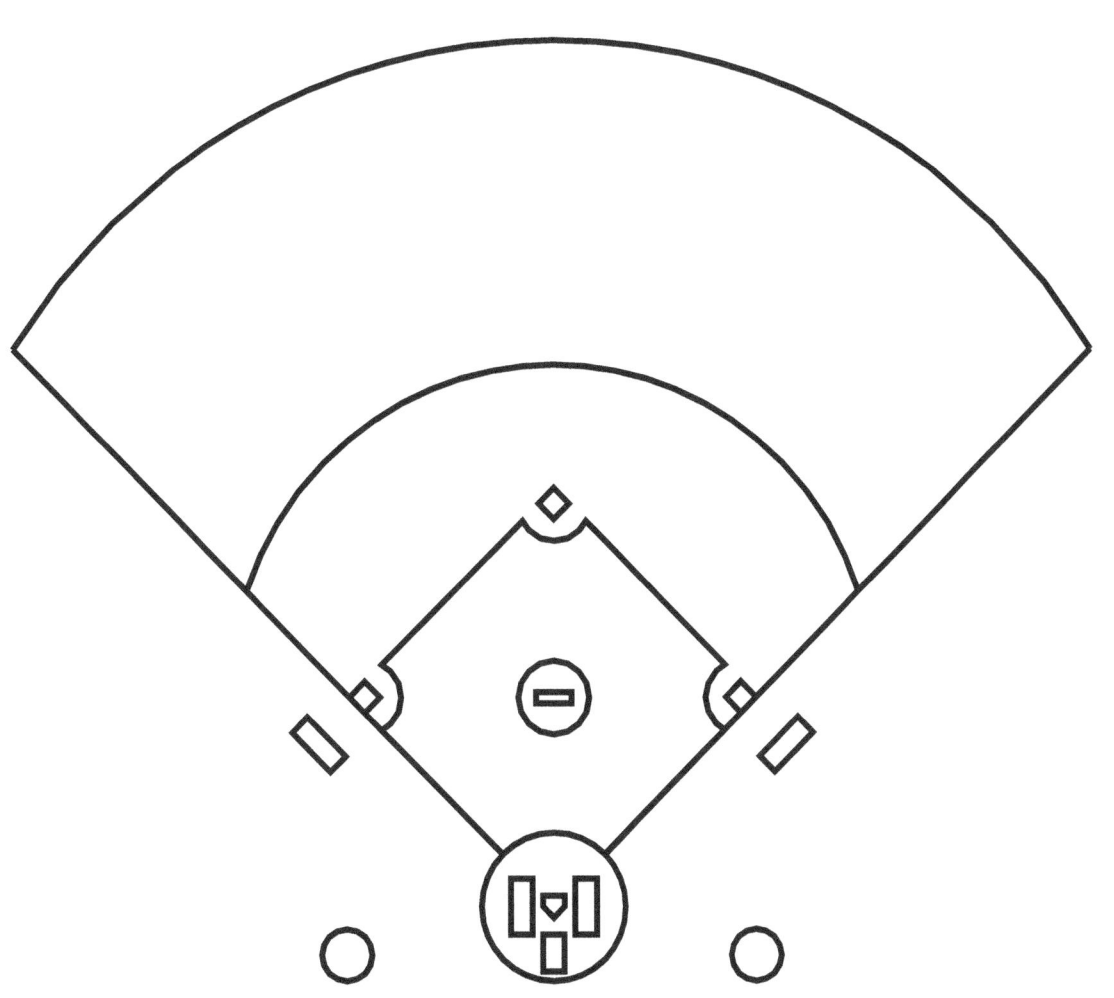

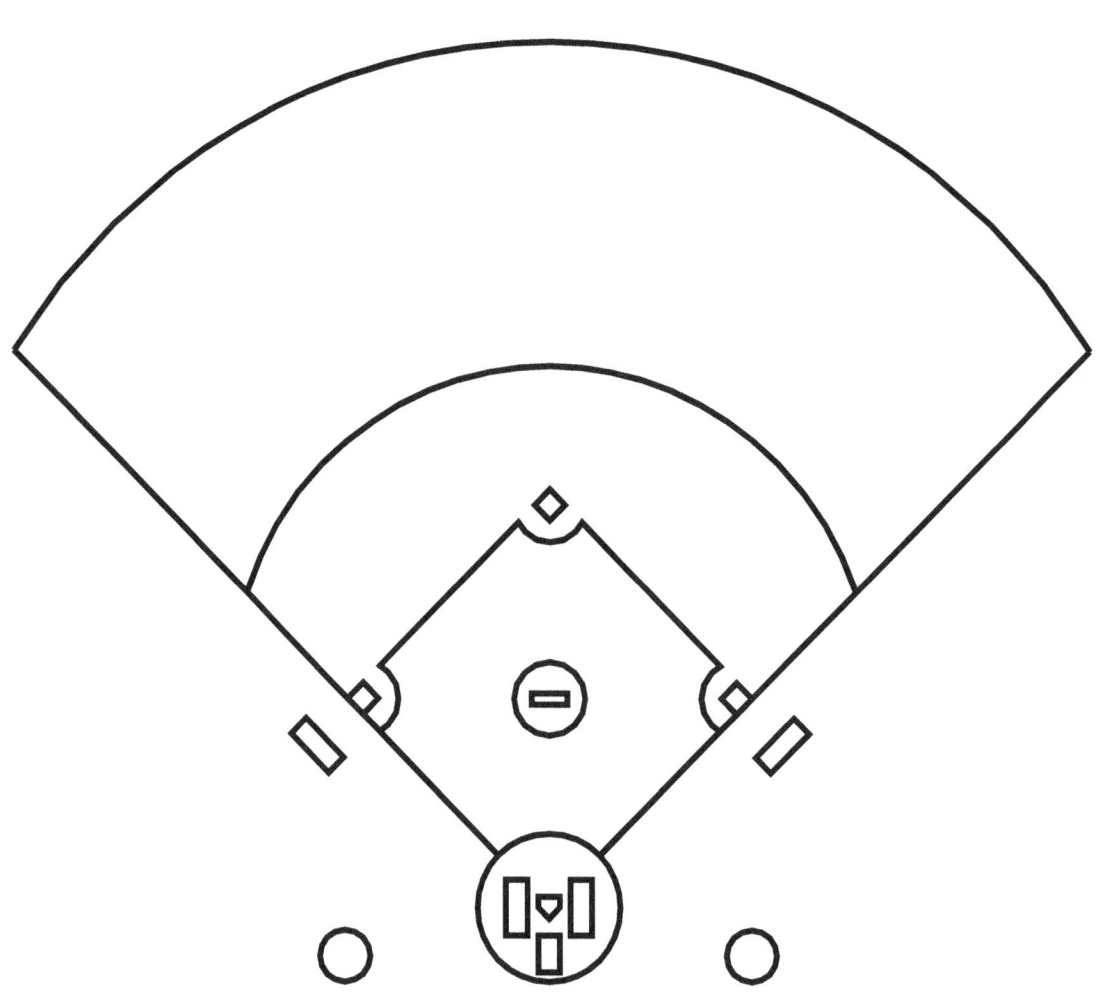

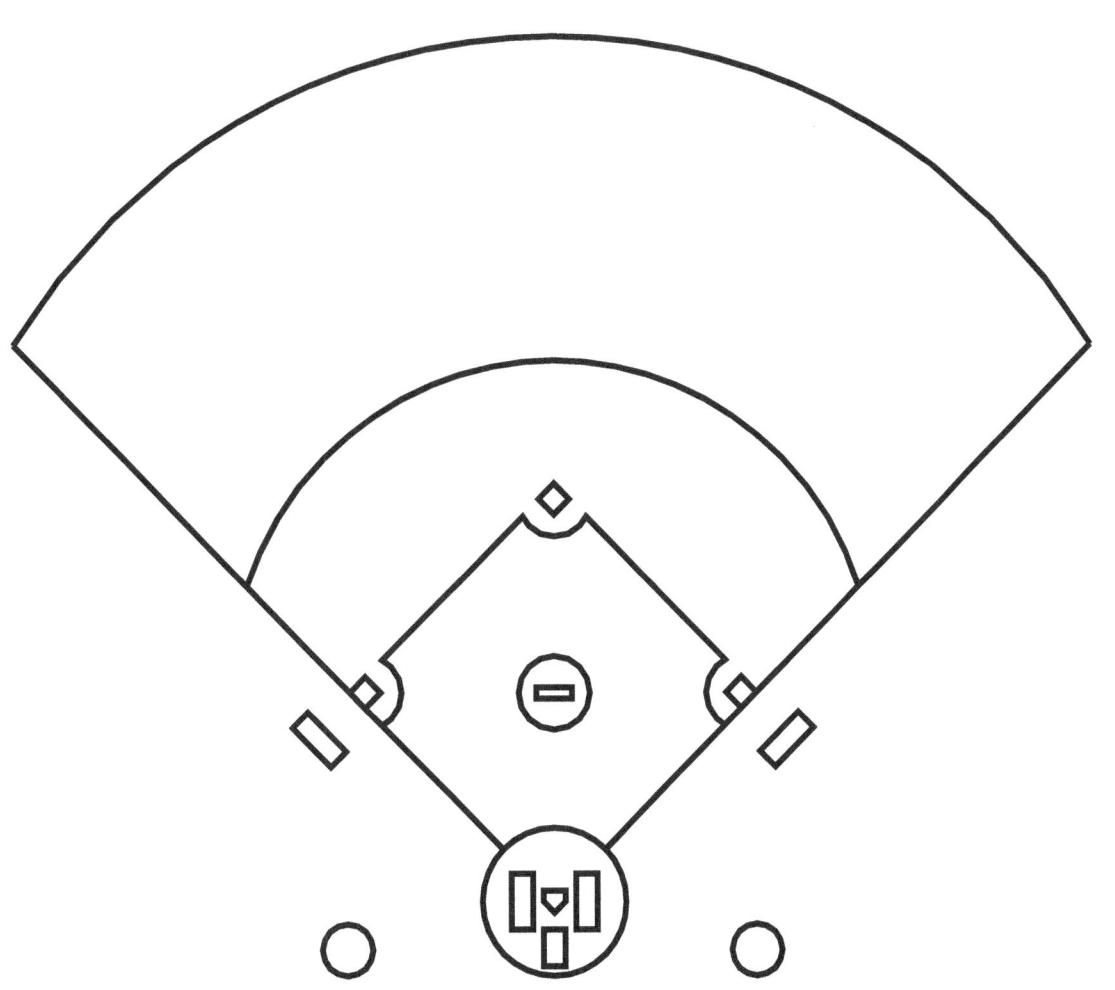

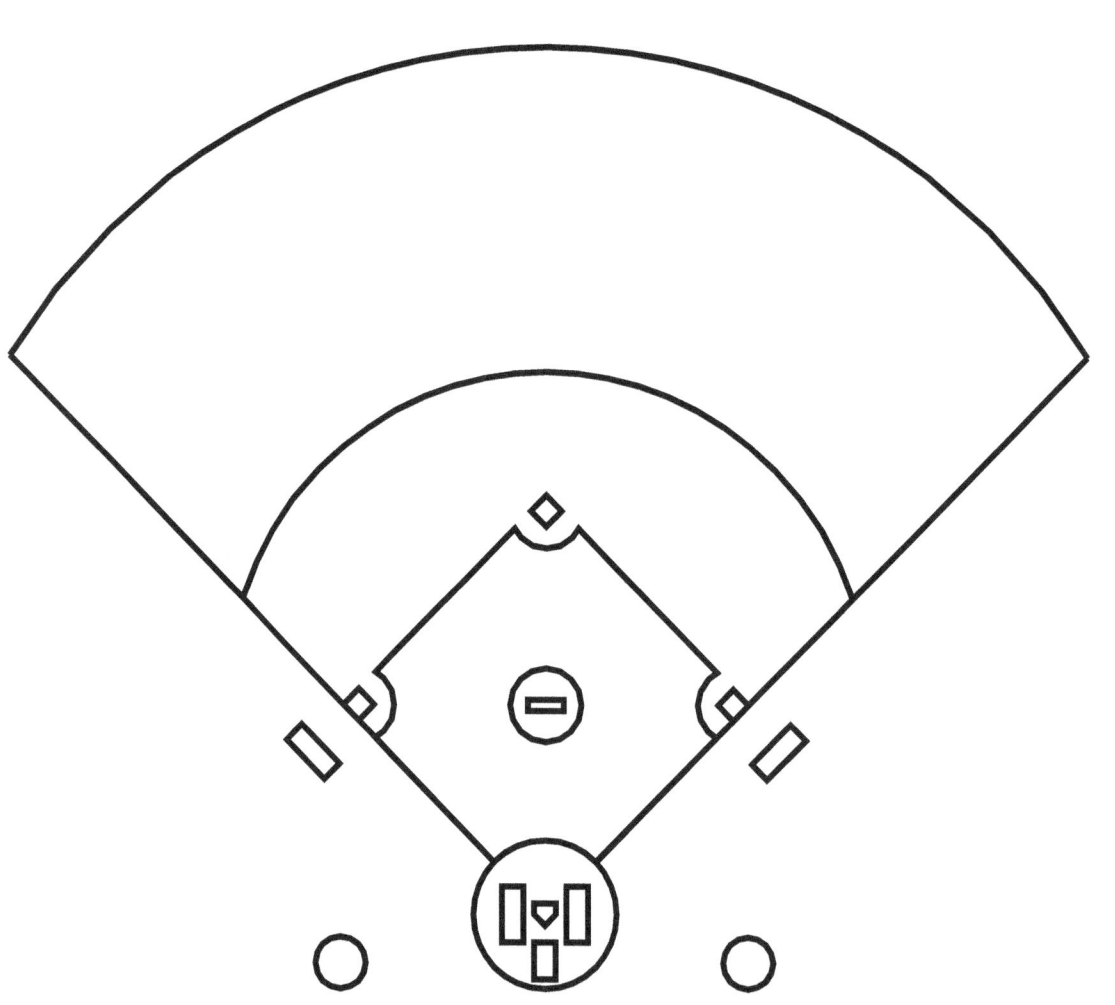

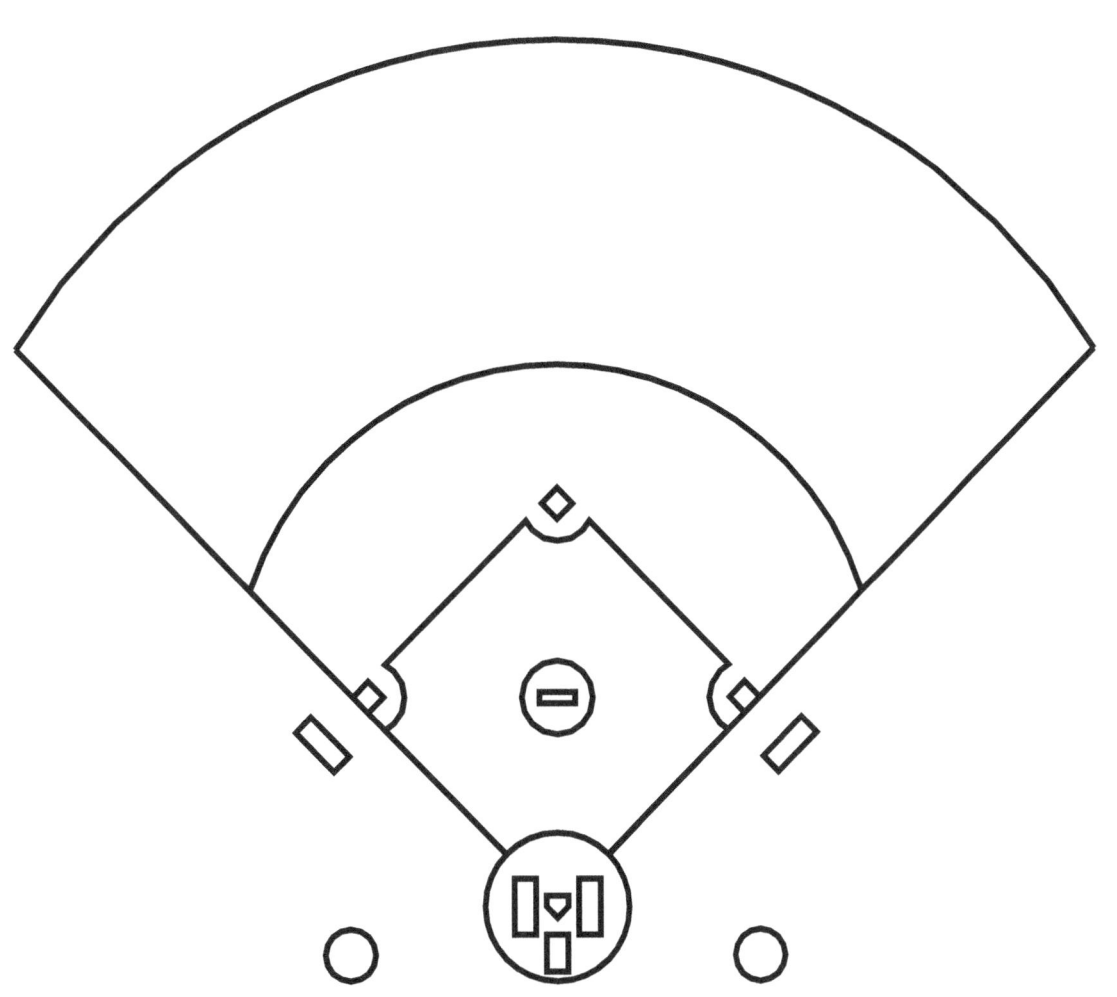

PRE-SEASON PRACTICE

Date:

Location:

My focus this week is:

Coach's focus this week is:

Skills I need to work on this week are:

I showed good sportsmanship this week by:

How I feel starting out:

This week's practice notes:

PRACTICE DAY

Date:

Location:

My focus this week is:

Coach's focus this week is:

Skills I need to work on this week are:

I showed good sportsmanship this week by:

How I feel starting out:

This week's practice notes:

GAME DAY

Date:

Opponent:

Location:

My focus today is:

Coach's focus today is:

Skills I need to work on this week are:

I showed good sportsmanship today by:

How I feel starting out:

Game Day notes:

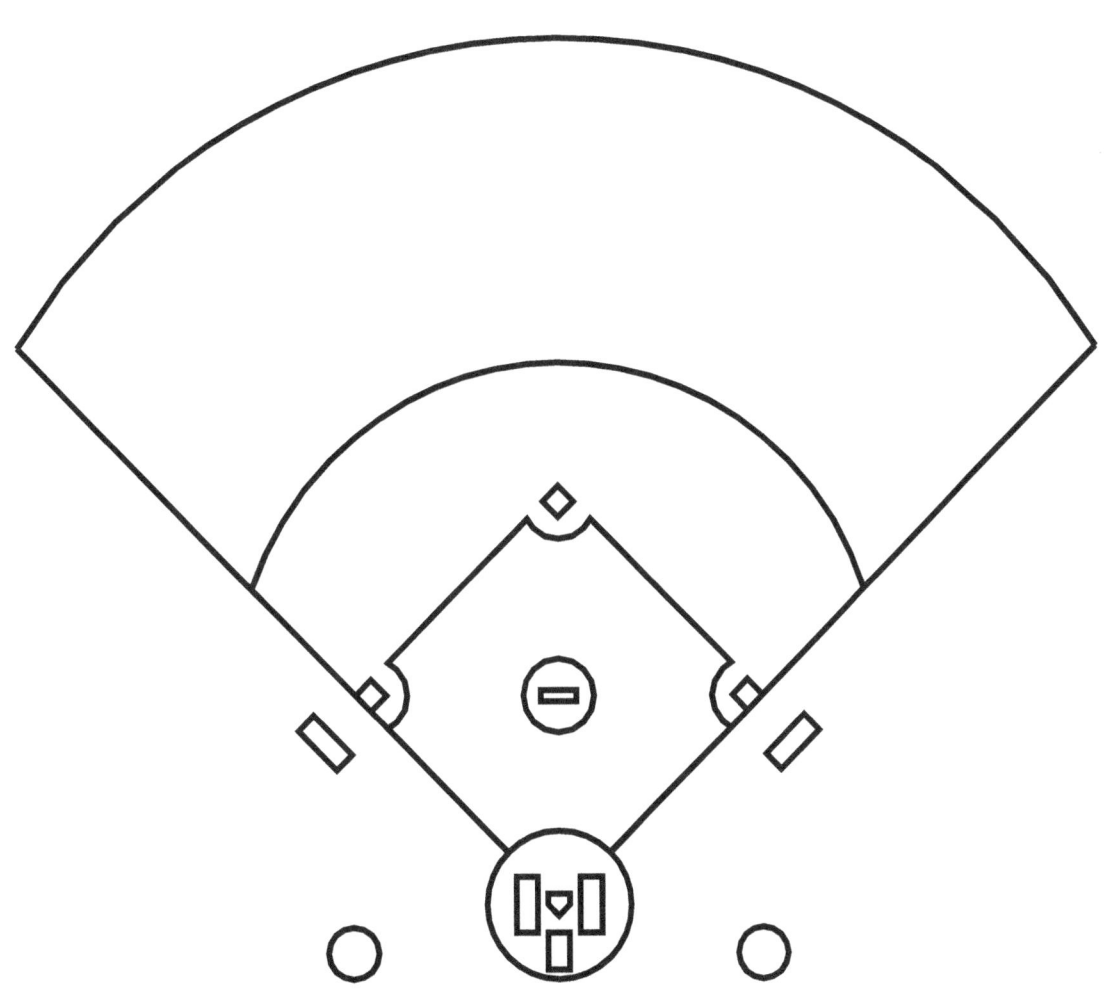

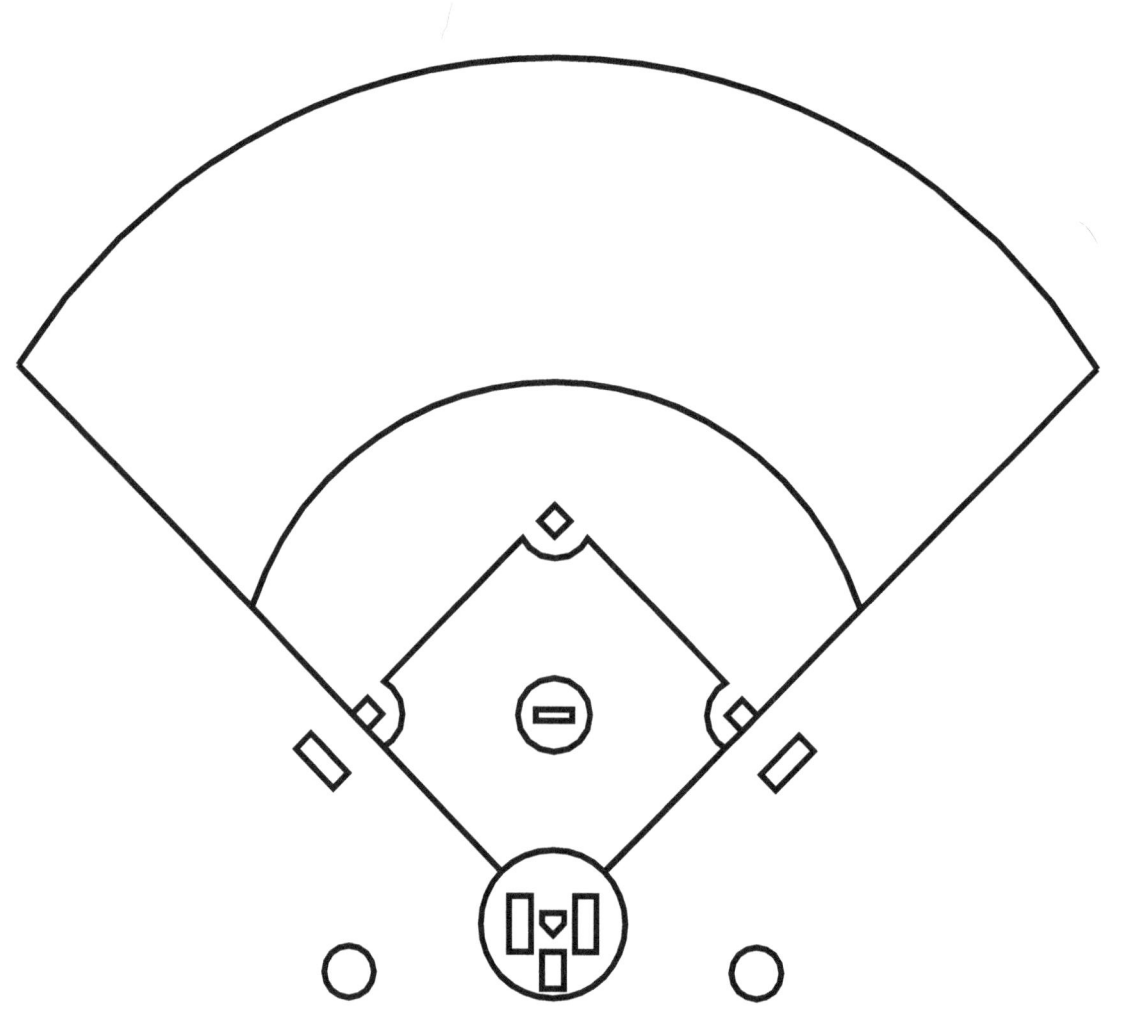

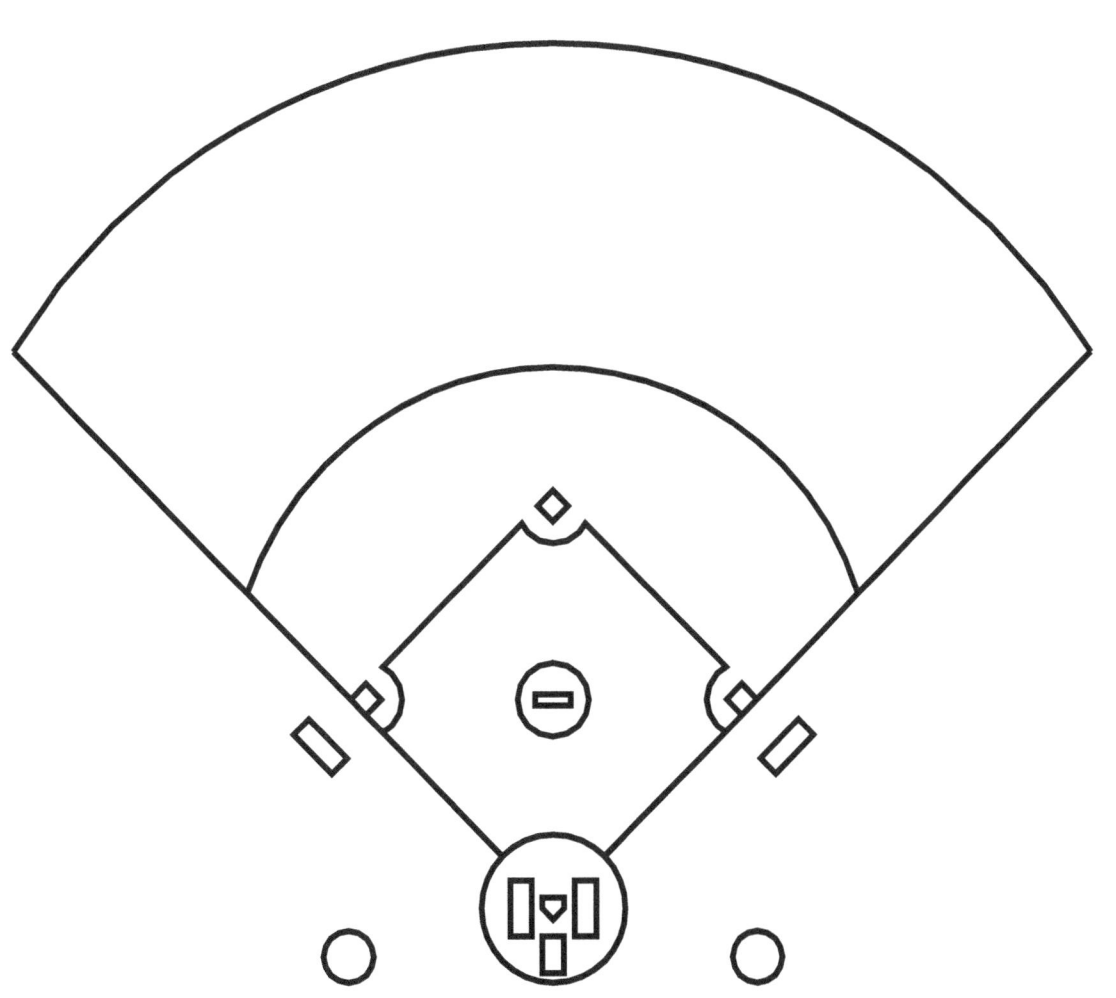

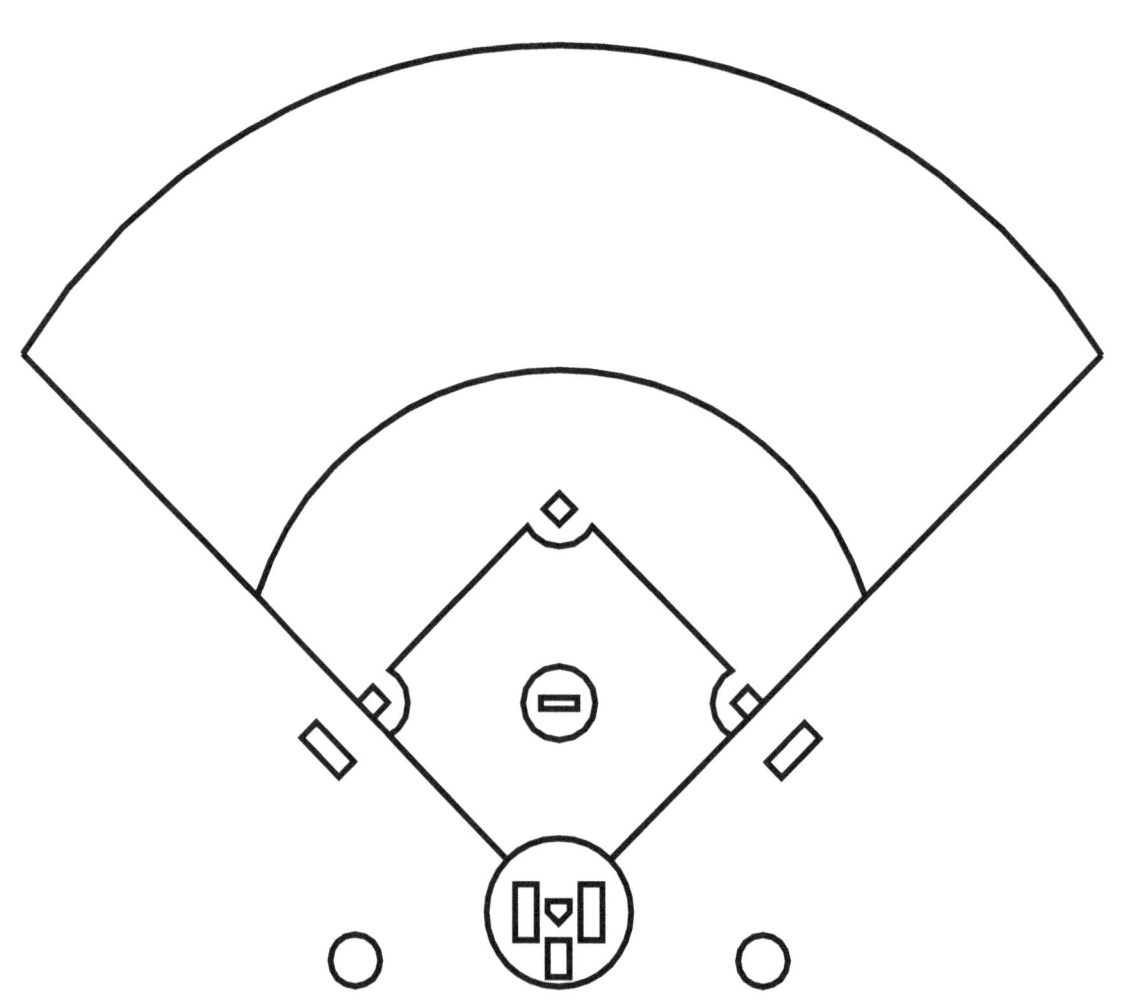

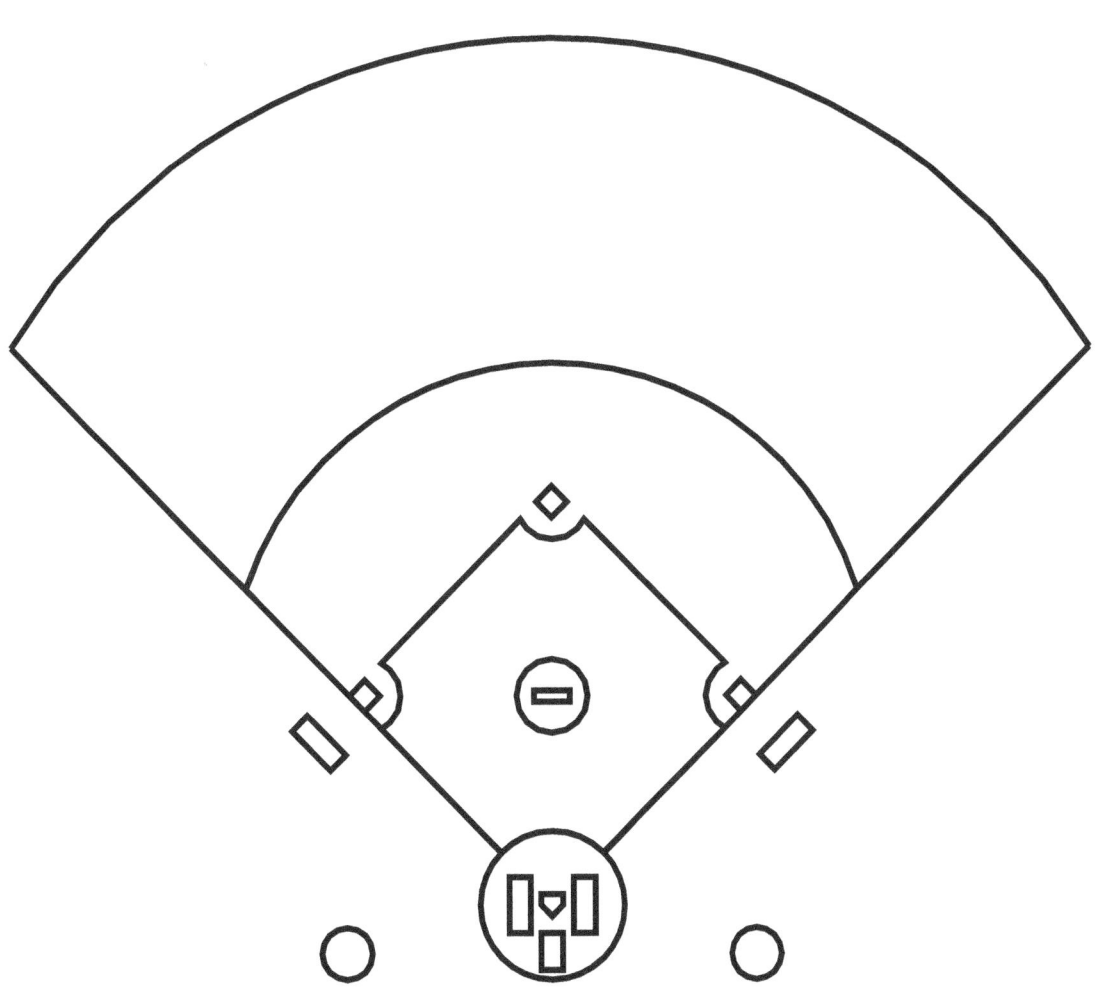

PRE-SEASON PRACTICE

Date:

Location:

My focus this week is:

Coach's focus this week is:

Skills I need to work on this week are:

I showed good sportsmanship this week by:

How I feel starting out:

This week's practice notes:

PRACTICE DAY

Date:

Location:

My focus this week is:

Coach's focus this week is:

Skills I need to work on this week are:

I showed good sportsmanship this week by:

How I feel starting out:

This week's practice notes:

GAME DAY

Date:

Opponent:

Location:

My focus today is:

Coach's focus today is:

Skills I need to work on this week are:

I showed good sportsmanship today by:

How I feel starting out:

Game Day notes:

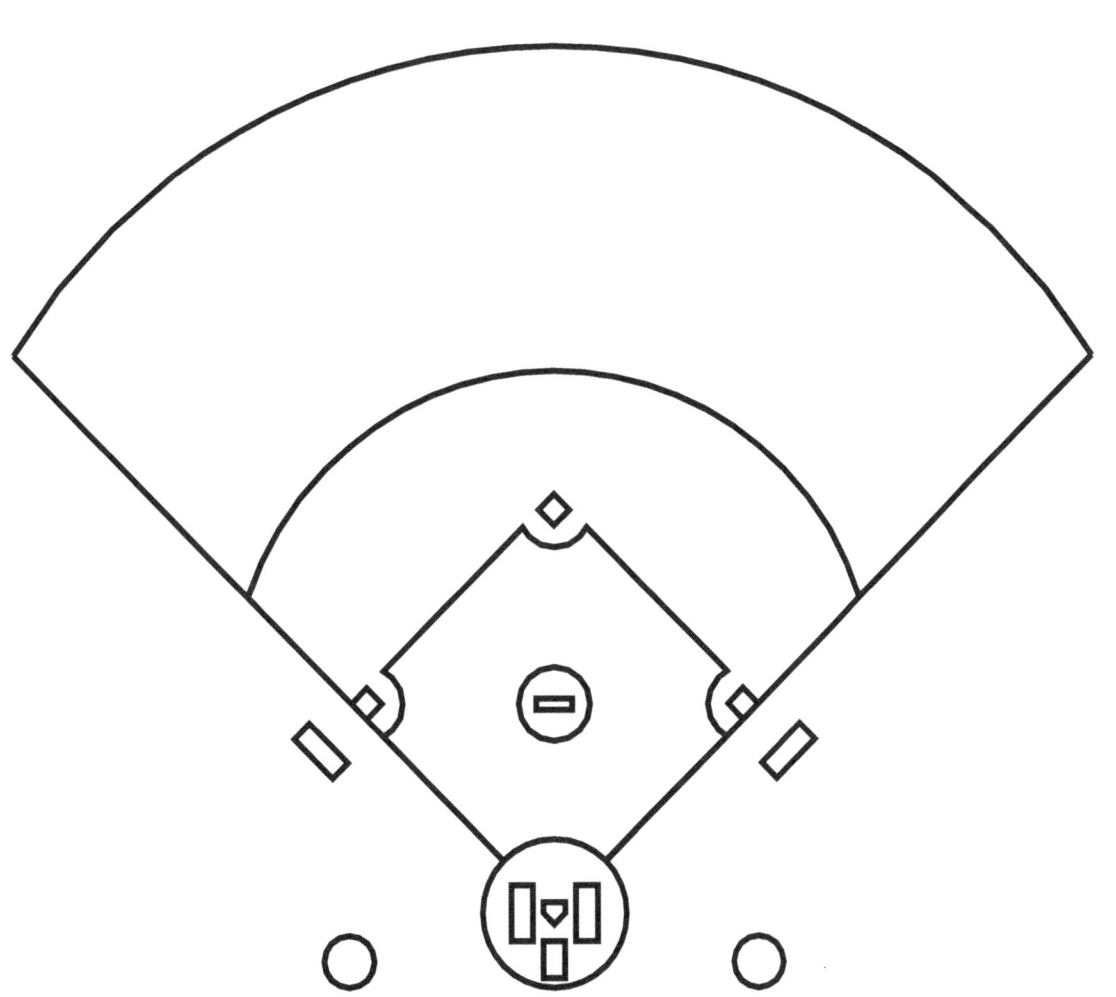

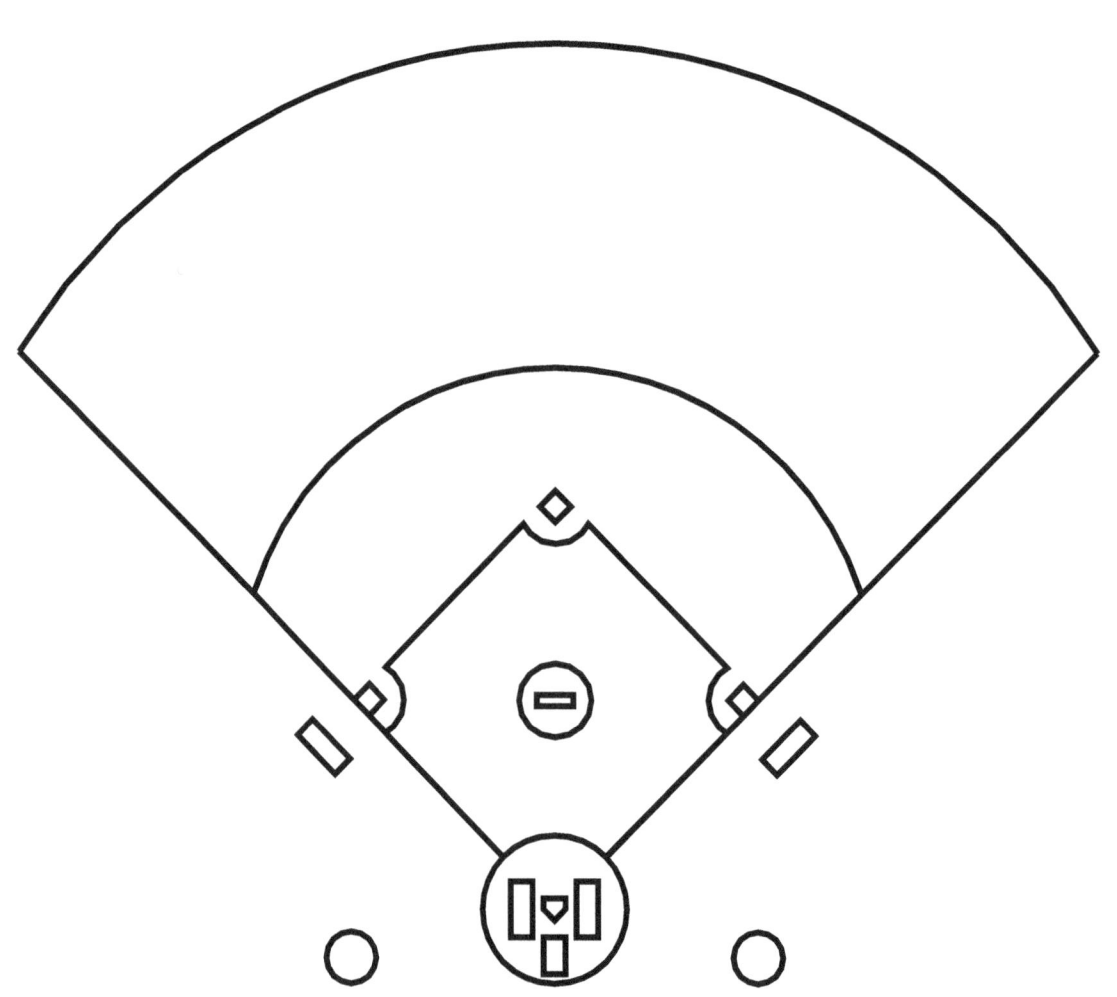

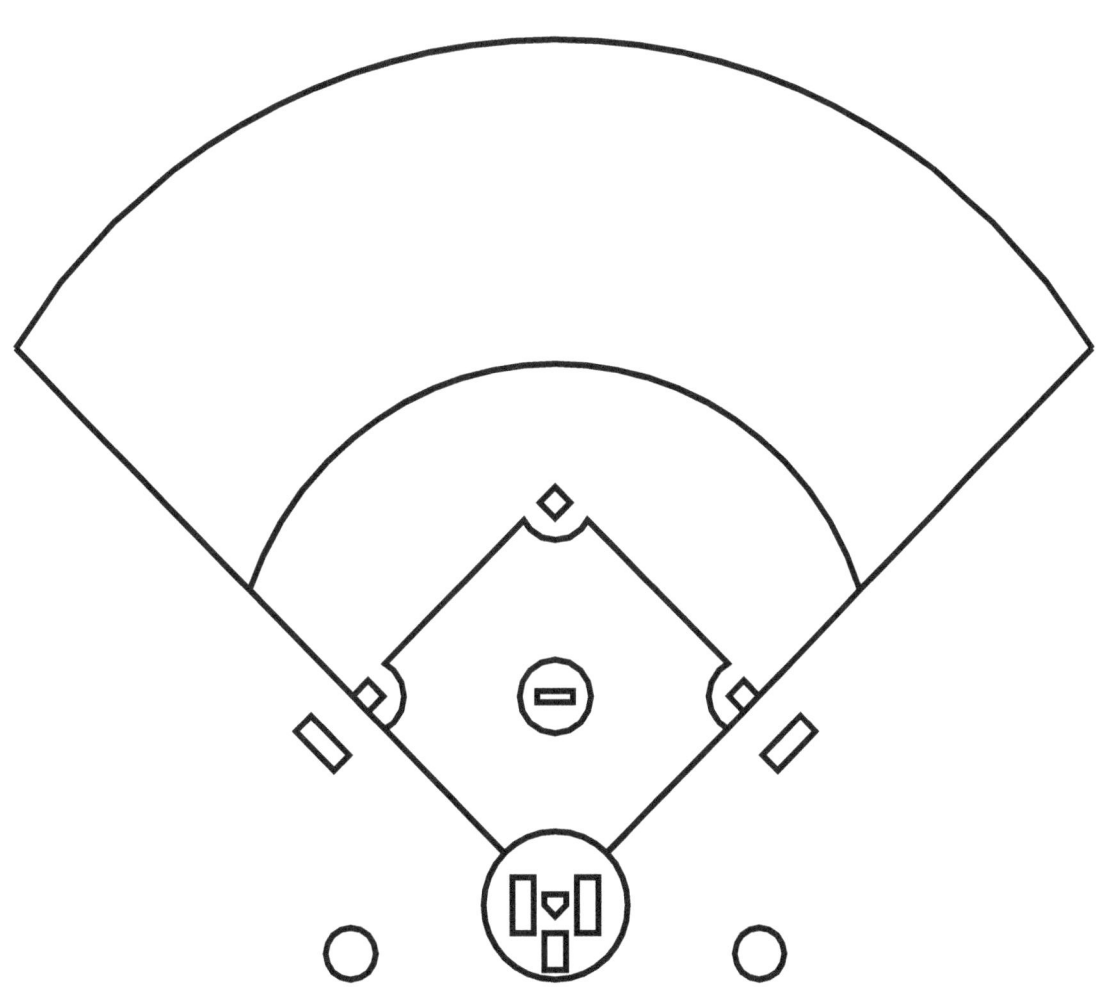

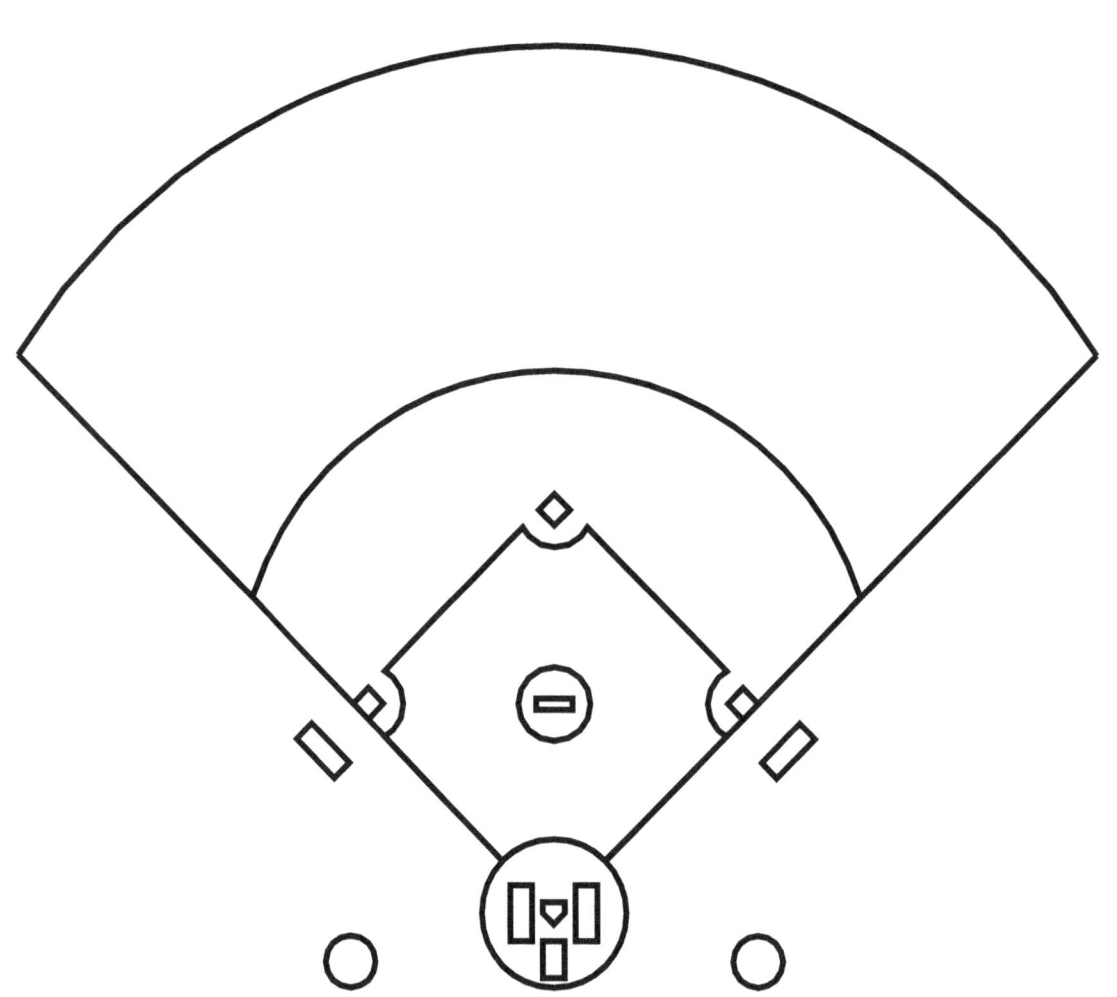

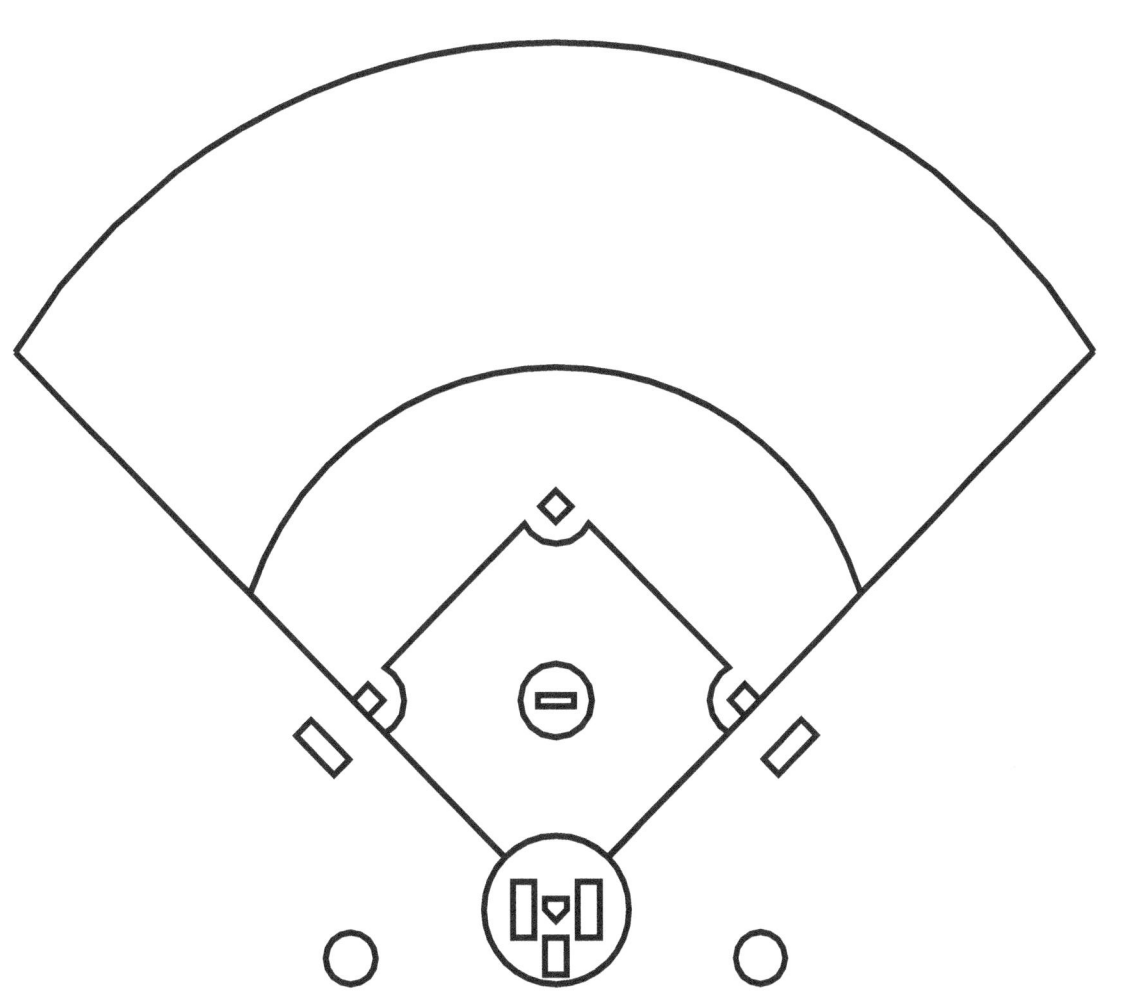

PRE-SEASON PRACTICE

Date:

Location:

My focus this week is:

Coach's focus this week is:

Skills I need to work on this week are:

I showed good sportsmanship this week by:

How I feel starting out:

This week's practice notes:

PRACTICE DAY

Date:

Location:

My focus this week is:

Coach's focus this week is:

Skills I need to work on this week are:

I showed good sportsmanship this week by:

How I feel starting out:

This week's practice notes:

GAME DAY

Date:

Opponent:

Location:

My focus today is:

Coach's focus today is:

Skills I need to work on this week are:

I showed good sportsmanship today by:

How I feel starting out:

Game Day notes:

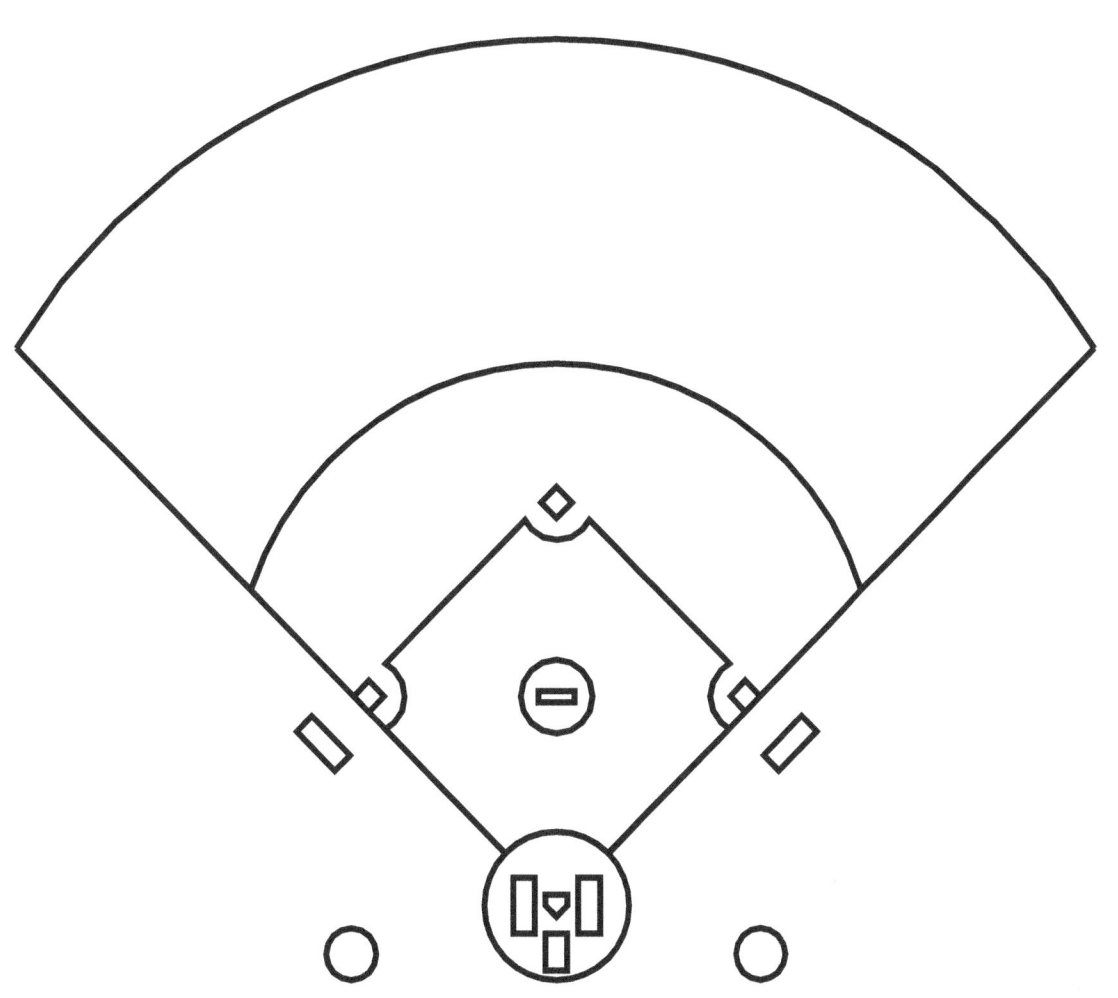

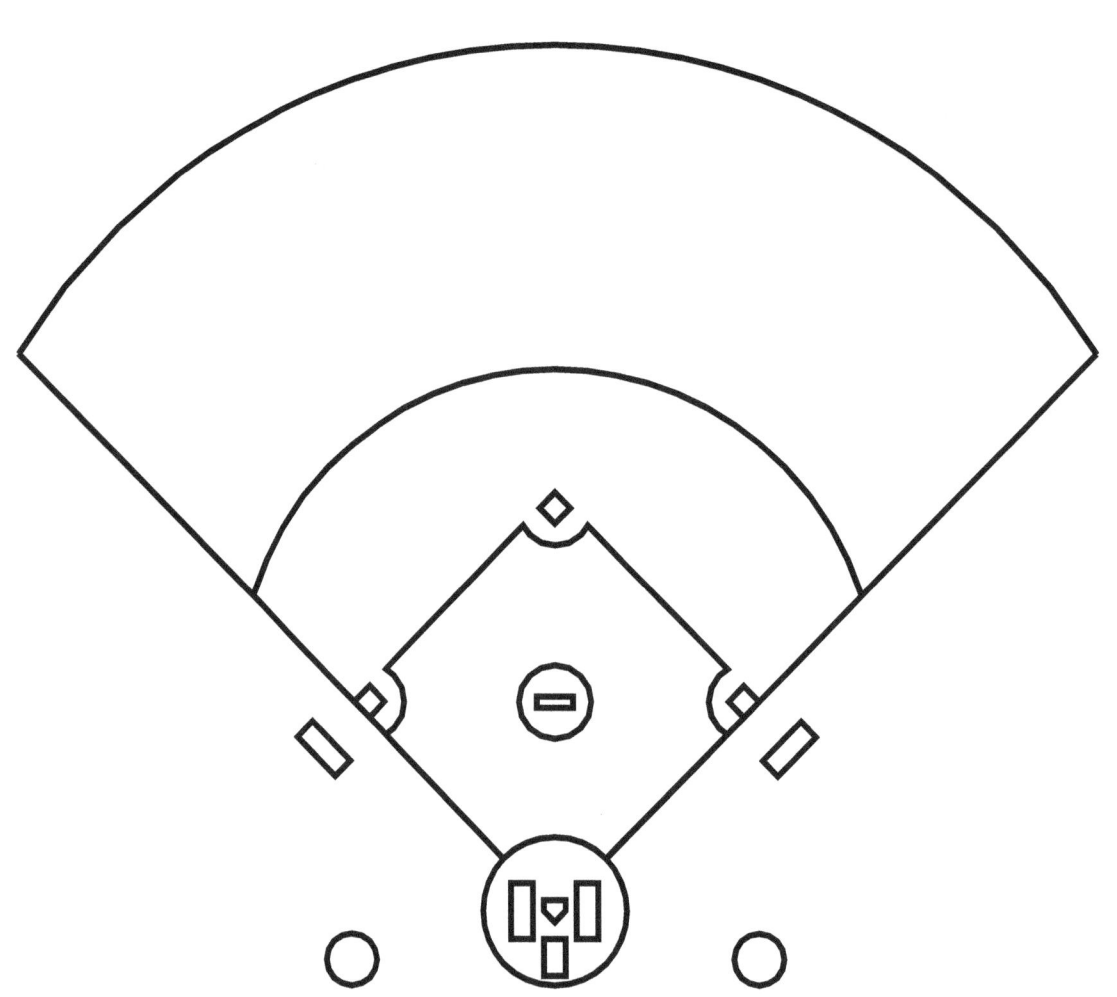

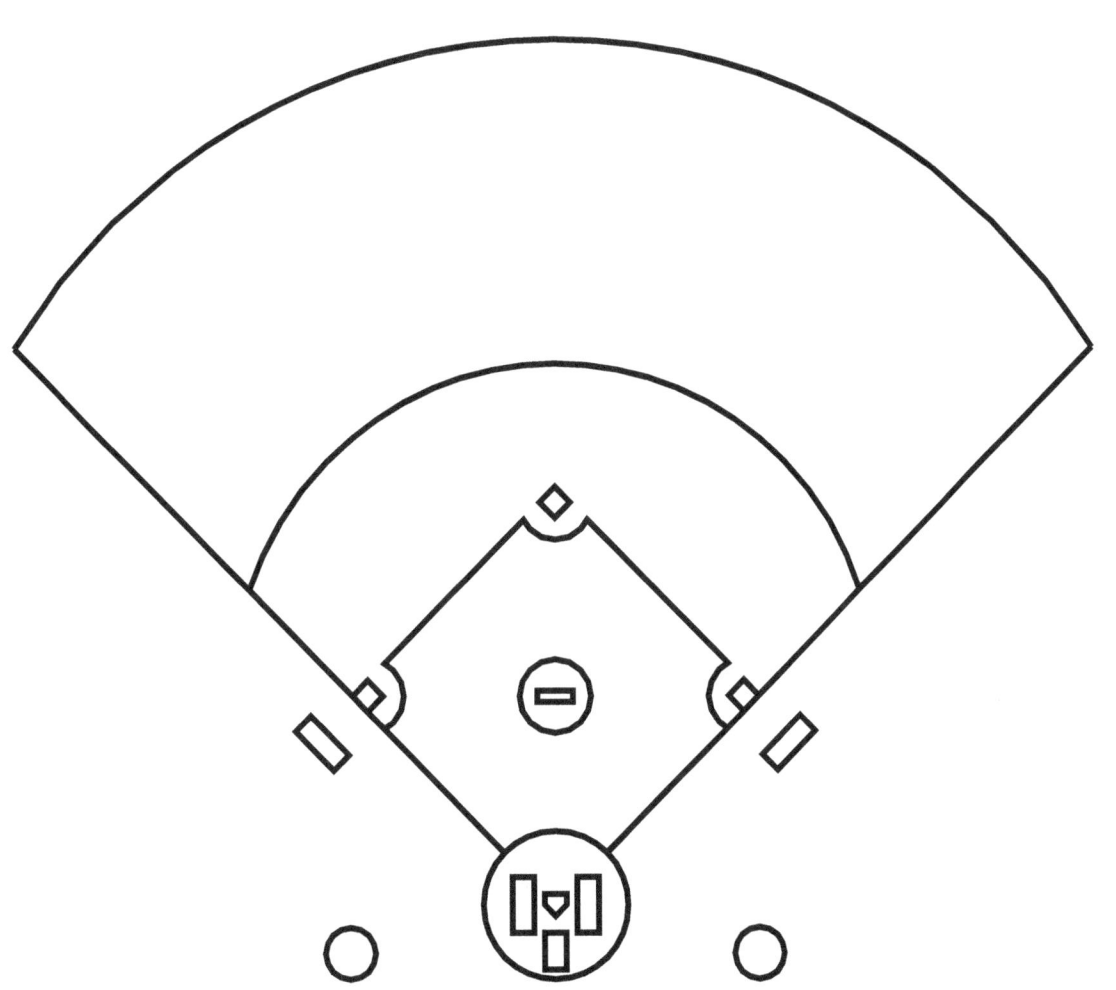

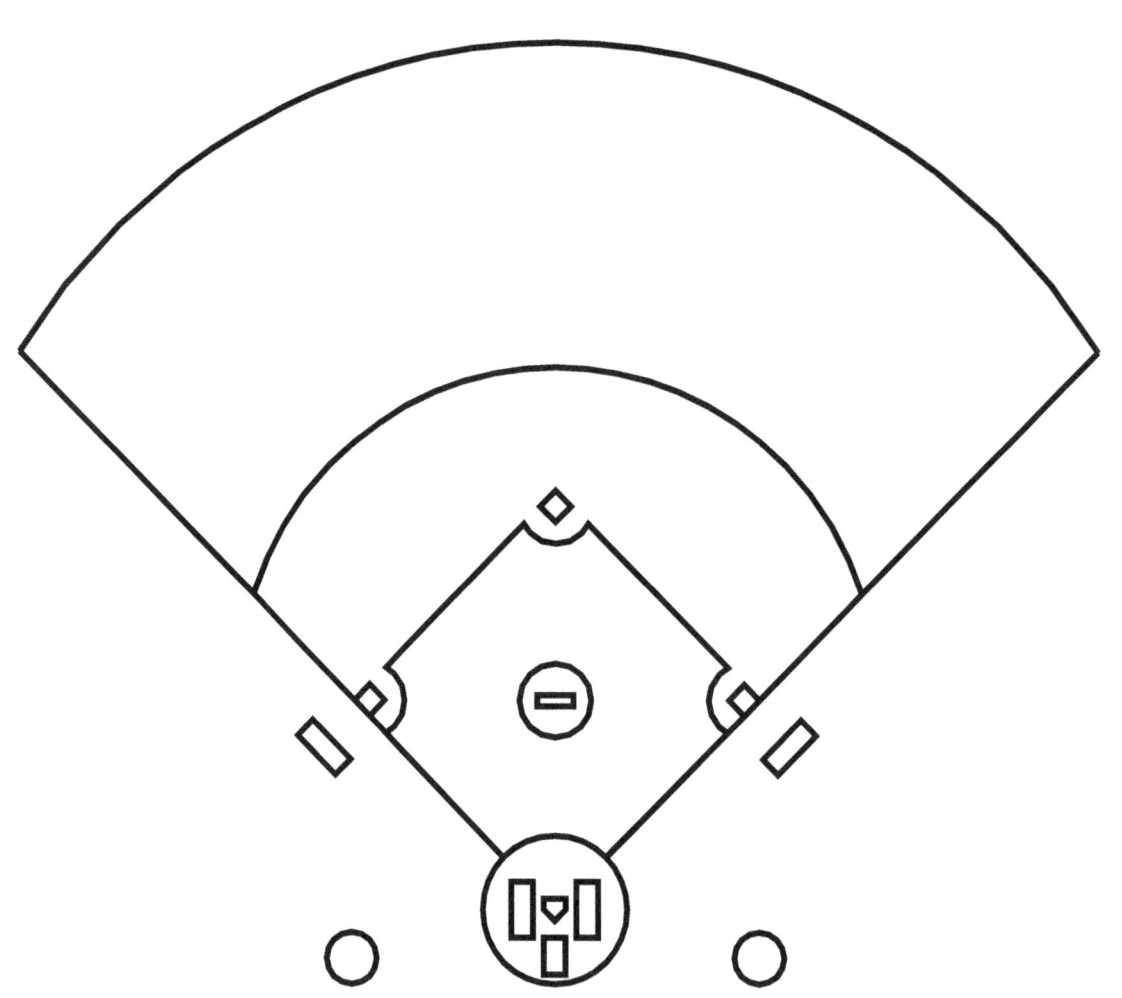

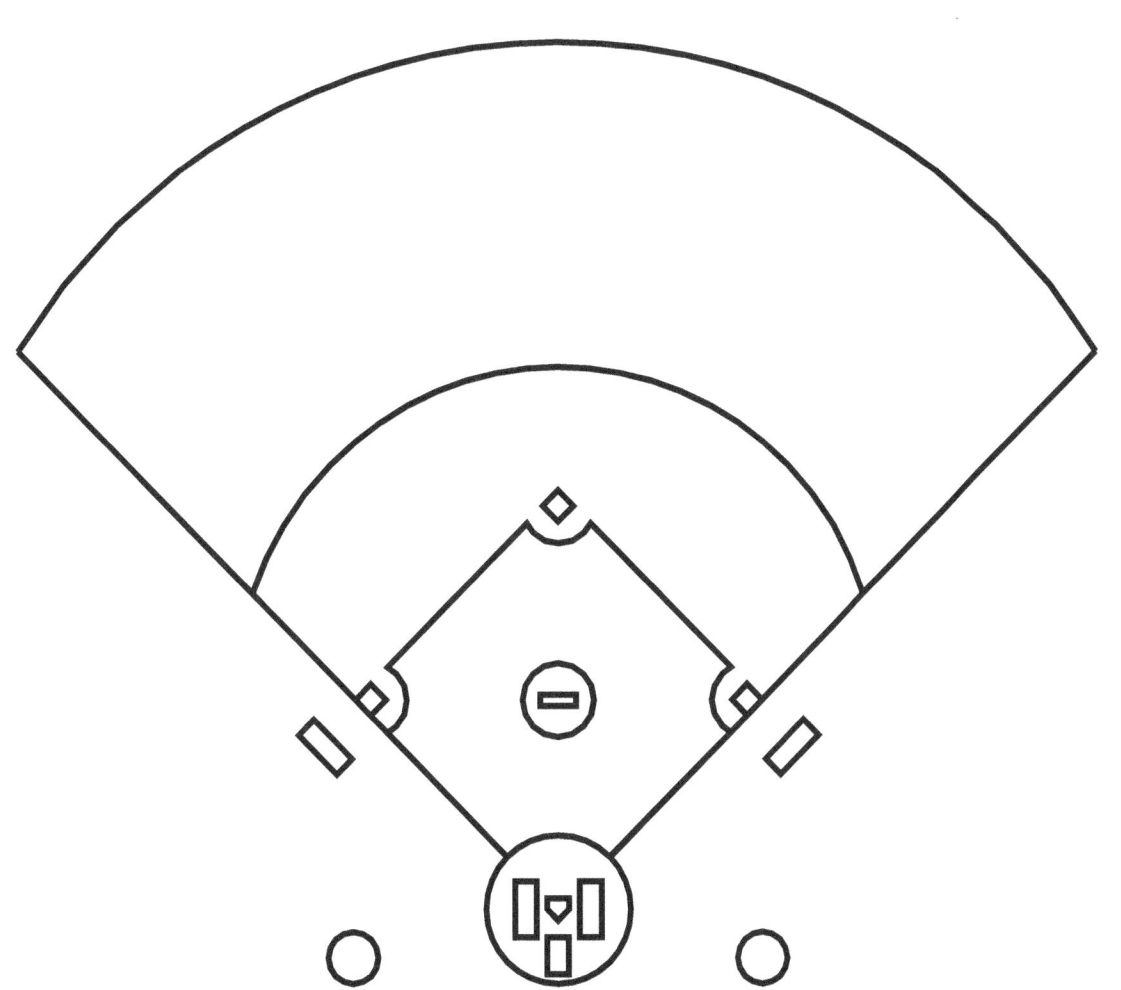

PRE-SEASON PRACTICE

Date:

Location:

My focus this week is:

Coach's focus this week is:

Skills I need to work on this week are:

I showed good sportsmanship this week by:

How I feel starting out:

This week's practice notes:

PRACTICE DAY

Date:

Location:

My focus this week is:

Coach's focus this week is:

Skills I need to work on this week are:

I showed good sportsmanship this week by:

How I feel starting out:

This week's practice notes:

GAME DAY

Date:

Opponent:

Location:

My focus today is:

Coach's focus today is:

Skills I need to work on this week are:

I showed good sportsmanship today by:

How I feel starting out:

Game Day notes:

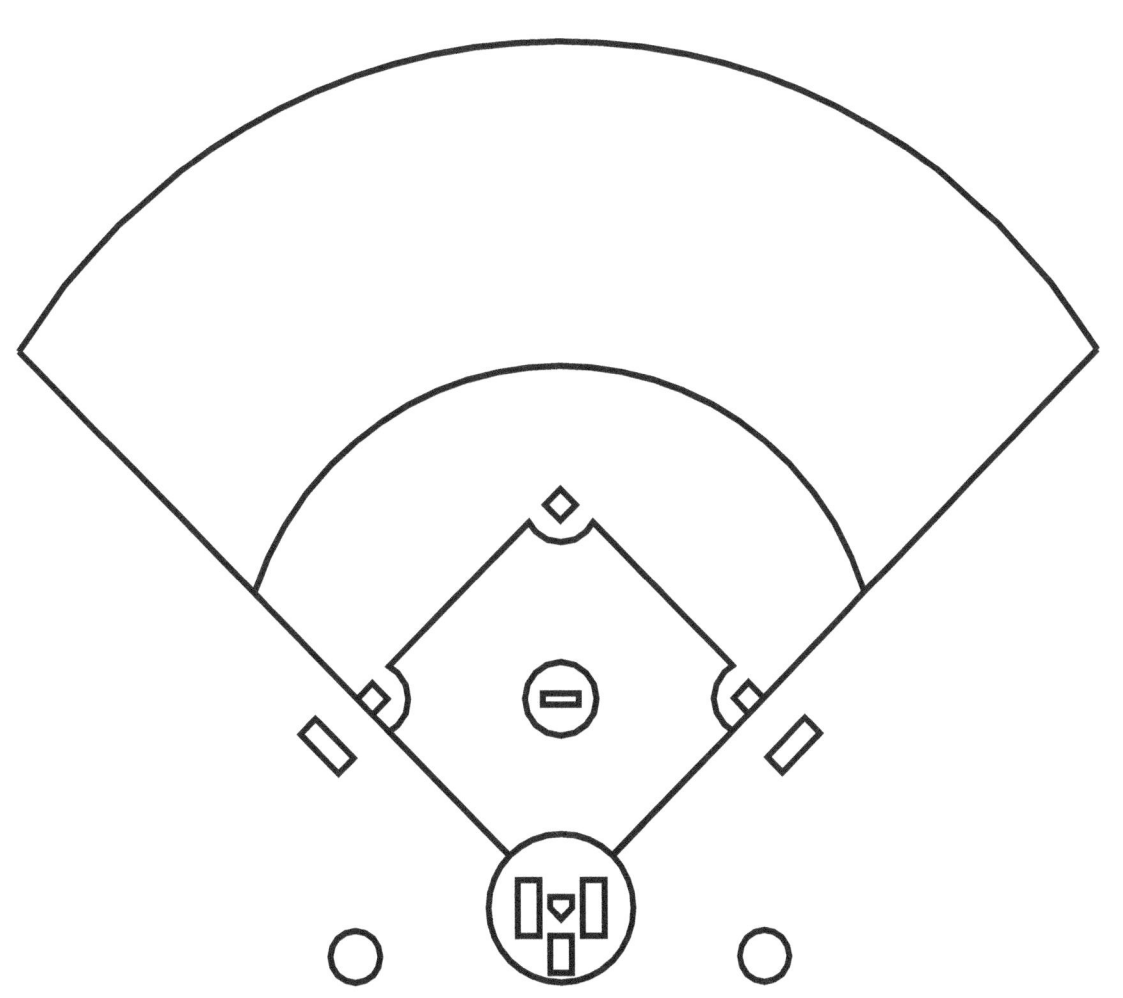

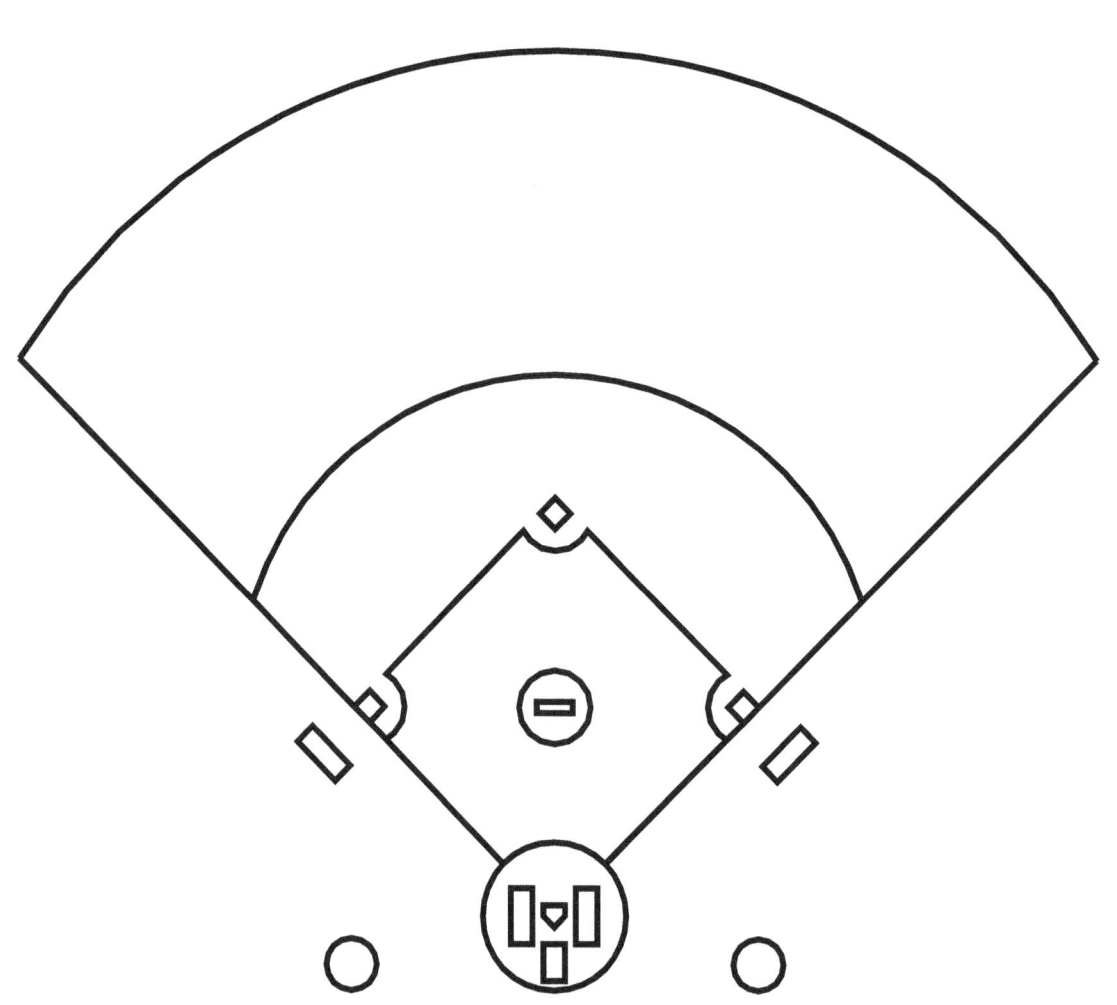

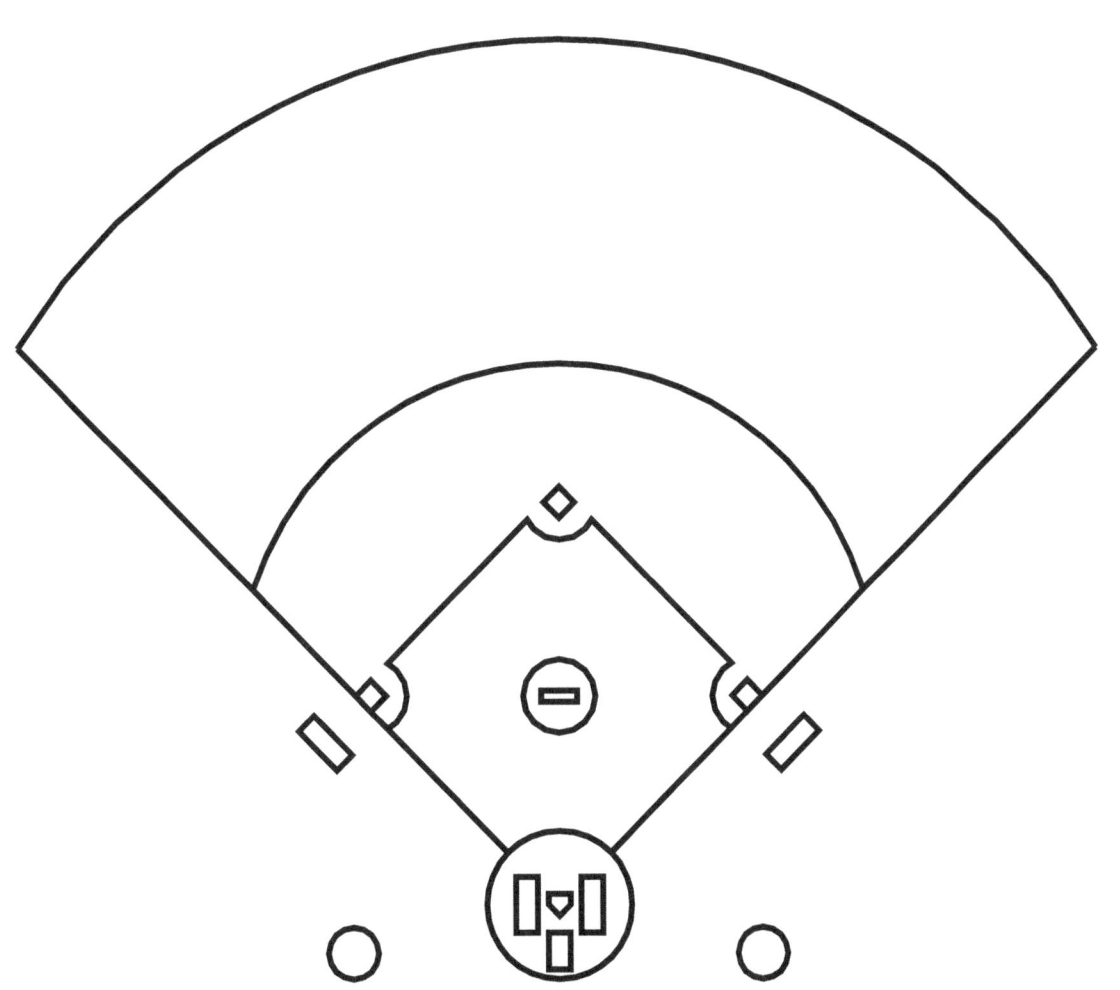

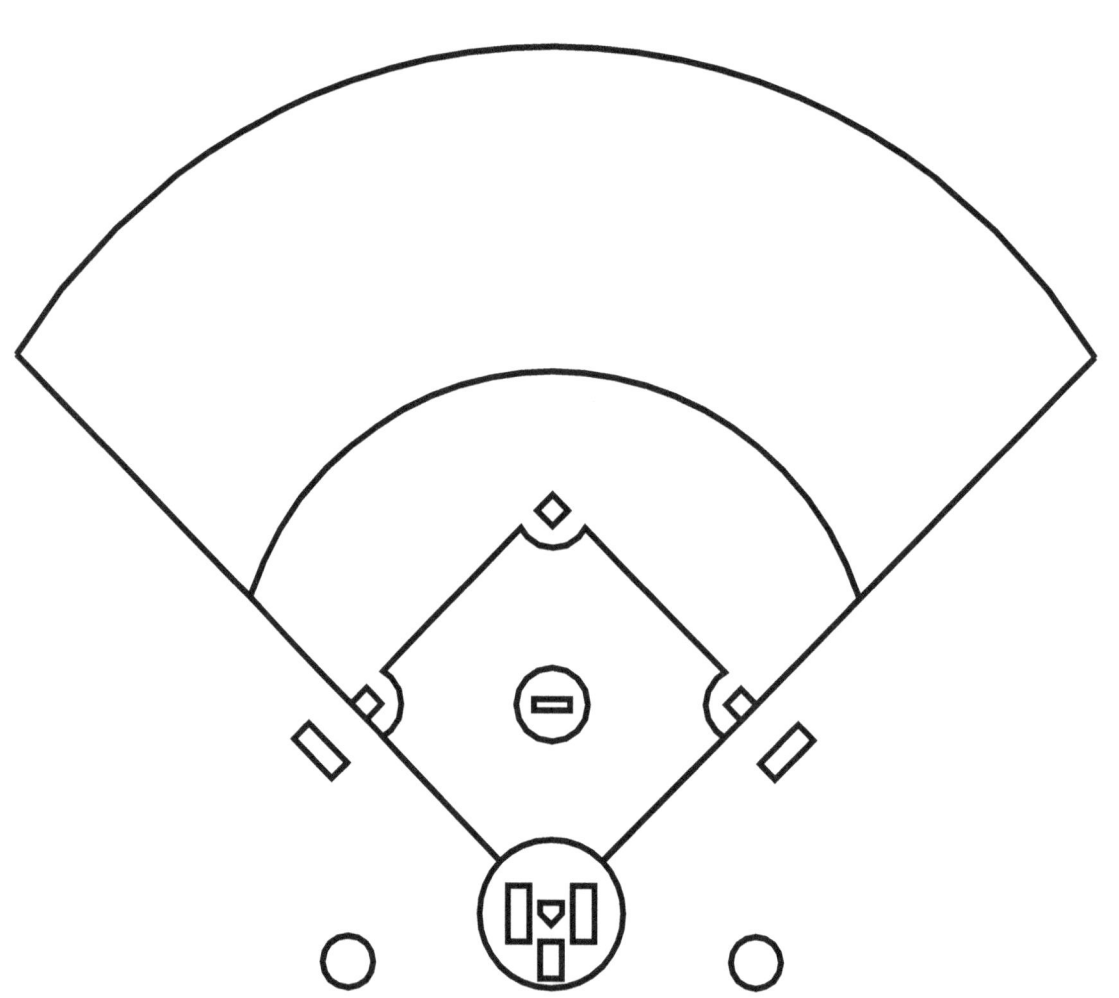

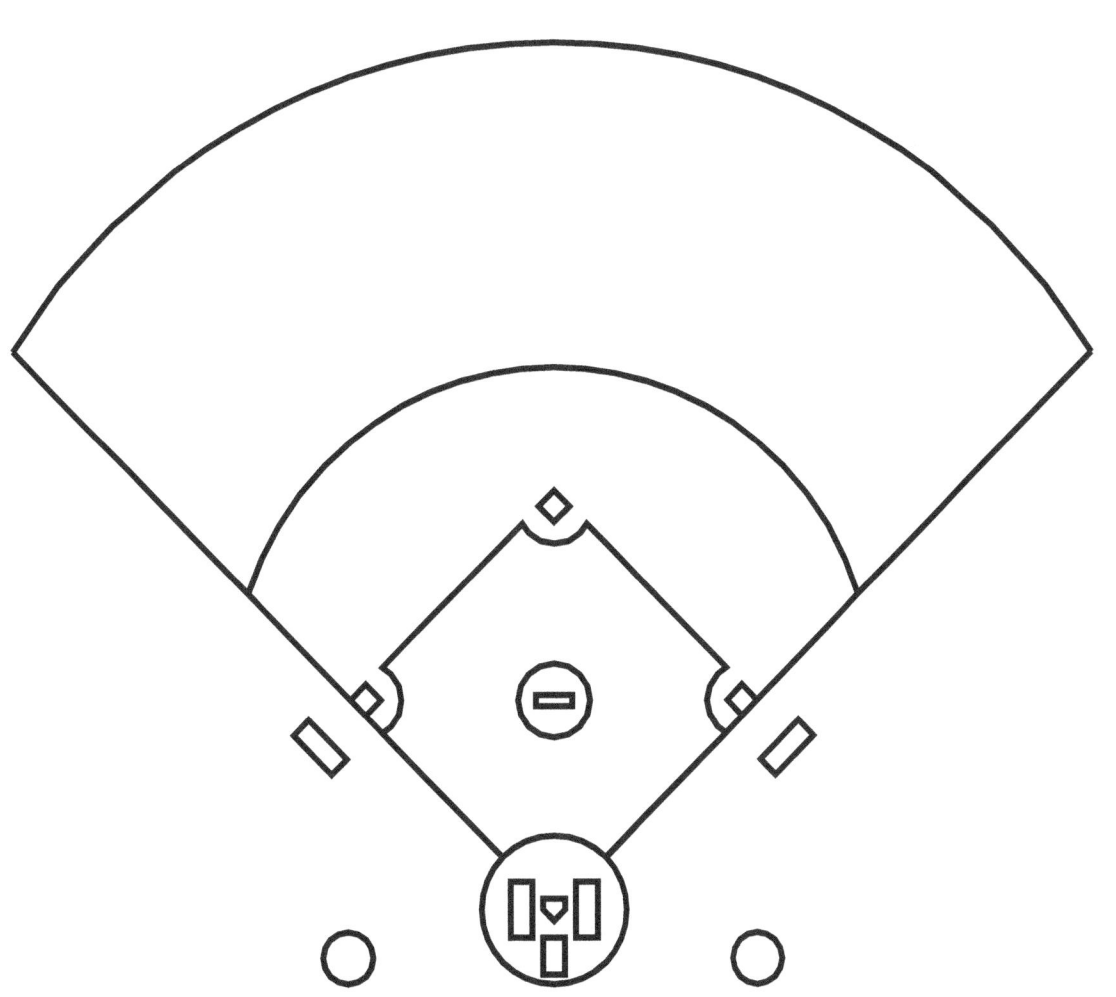

PRE-SEASON PRACTICE

Date:

Location:

My focus this week is:

Coach's focus this week is:

Skills I need to work on this week are:

I showed good sportsmanship this week by:

How I feel starting out:

This week's practice notes:

PRACTICE DAY

Date:

Location:

My focus this week is:

Coach's focus this week is:

Skills I need to work on this week are:

I showed good sportsmanship this week by:

How I feel starting out:

This week's practice notes:

GAME DAY

Date:

Opponent:

Location:

My focus today is:

Coach's focus today is:

Skills I need to work on this week are:

I showed good sportsmanship today by:

How I feel starting out:

Game Day notes:

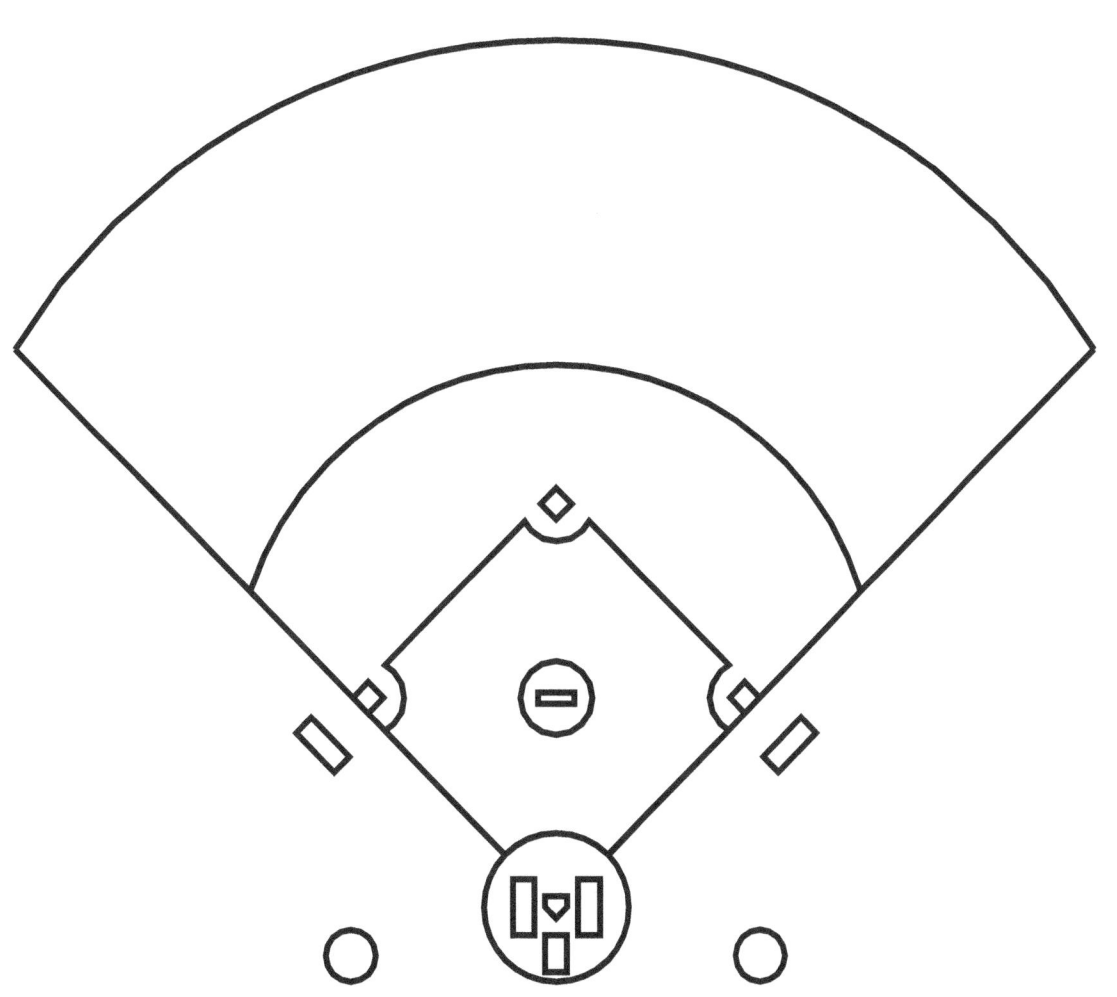

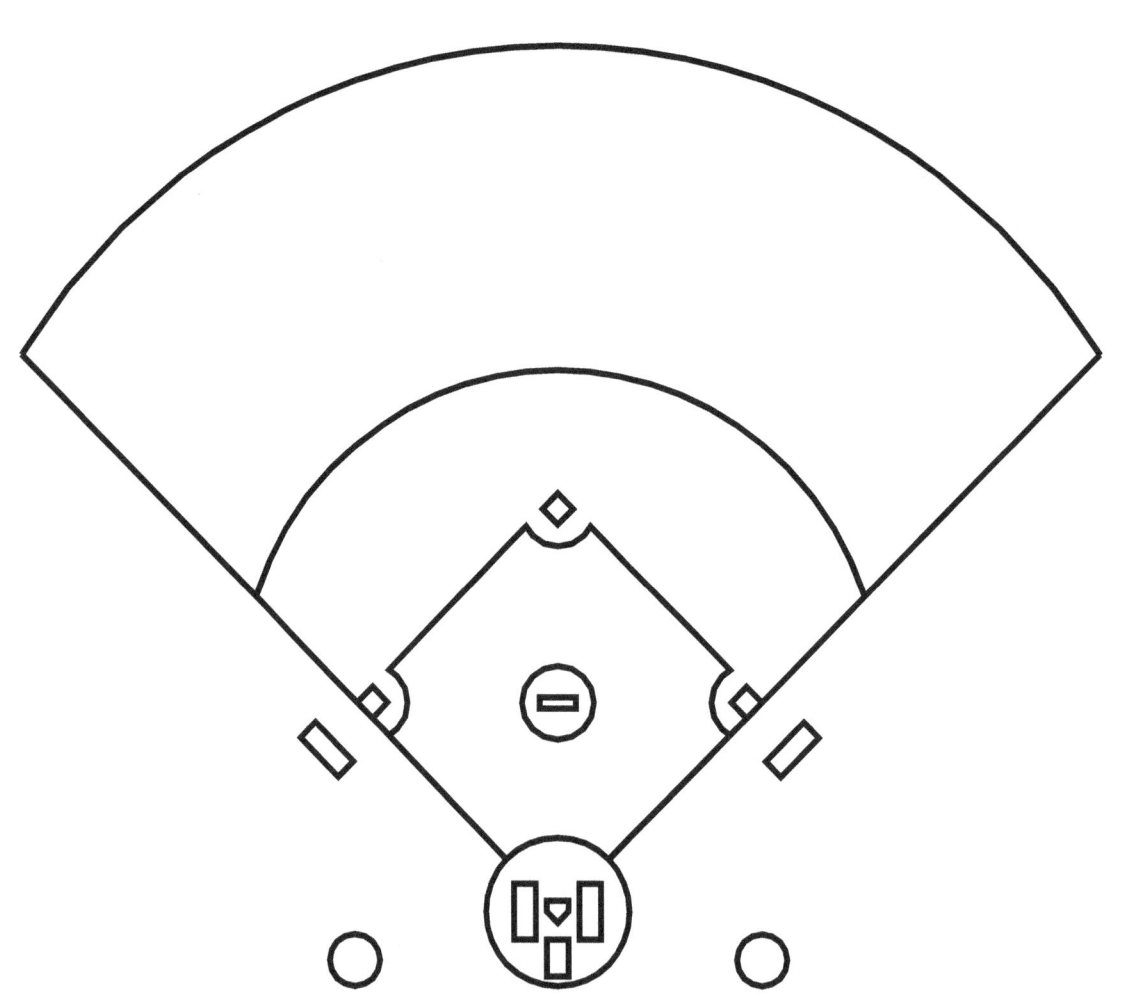

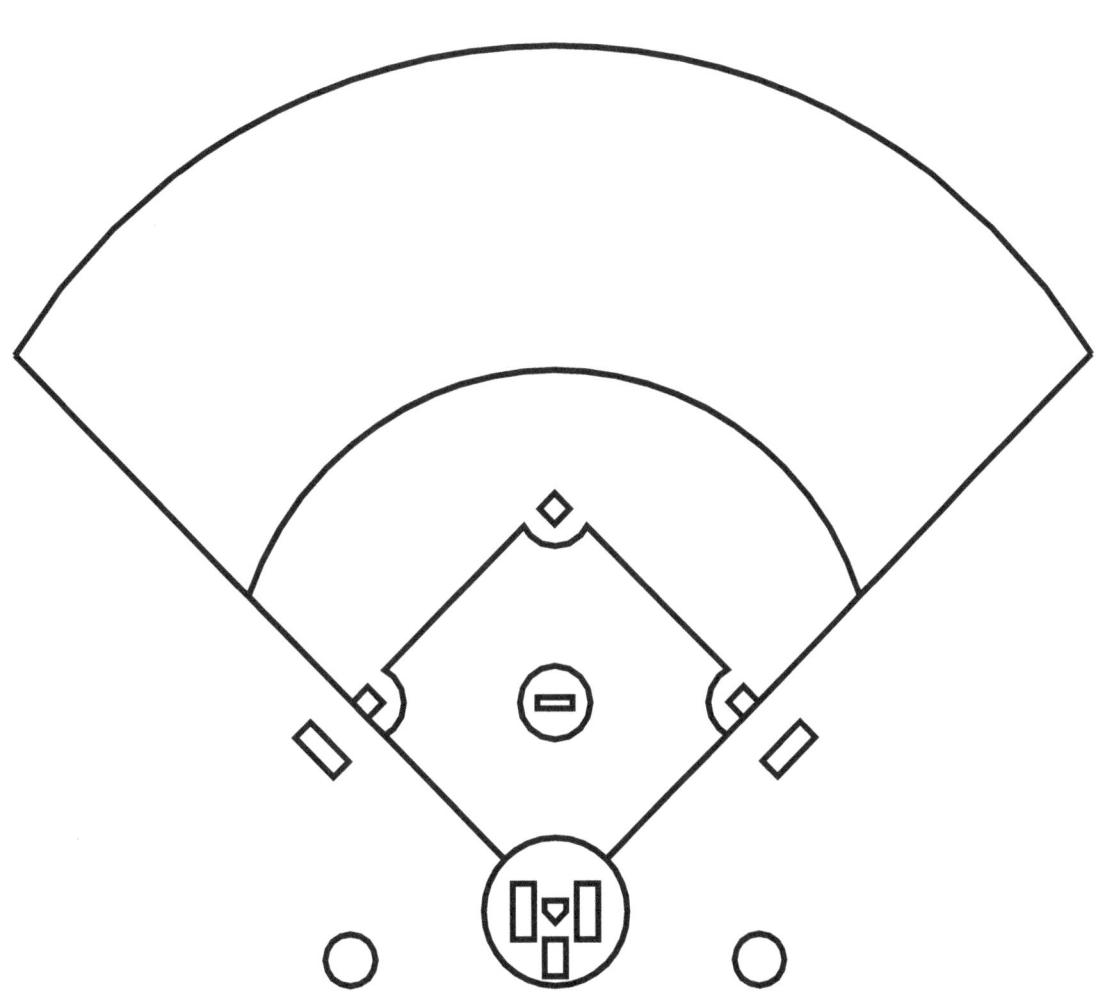

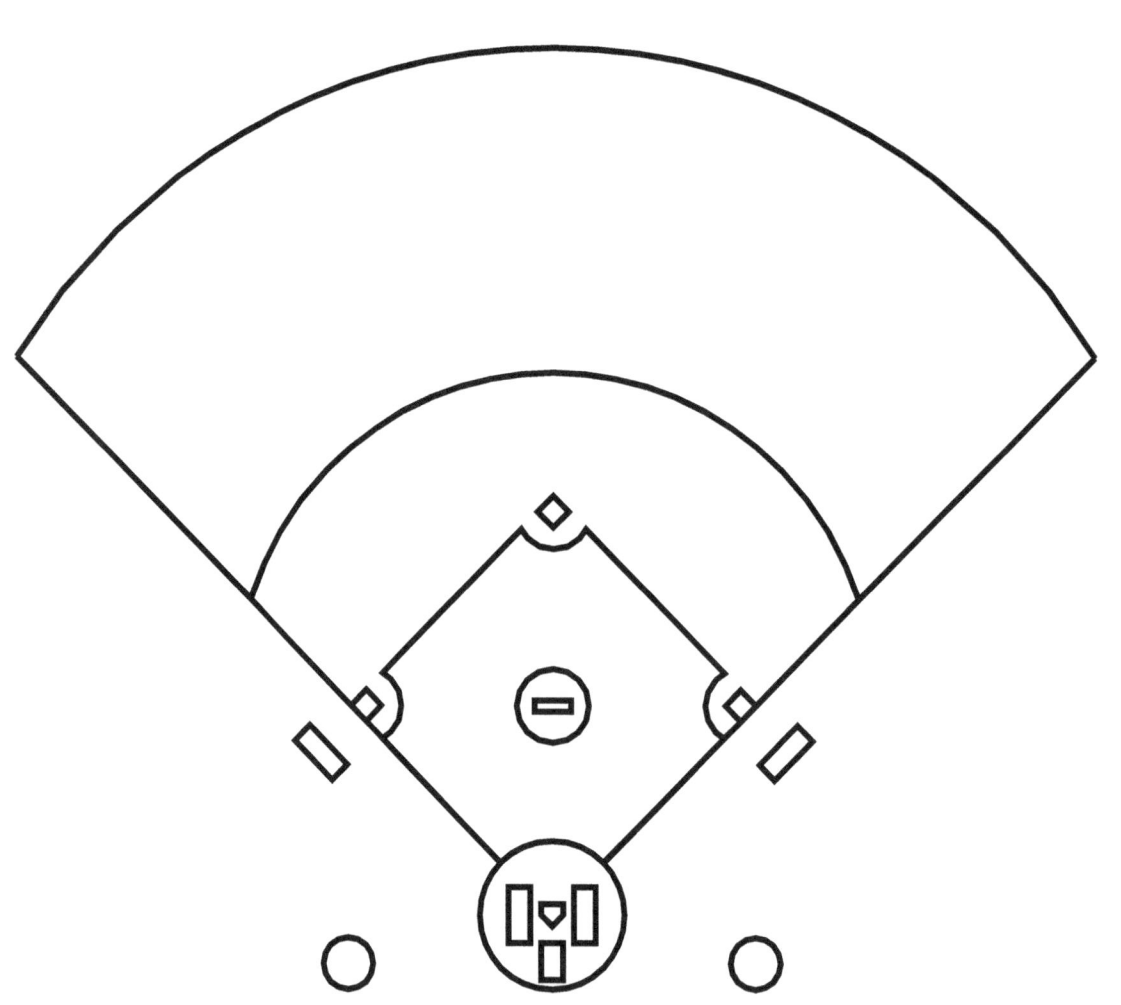

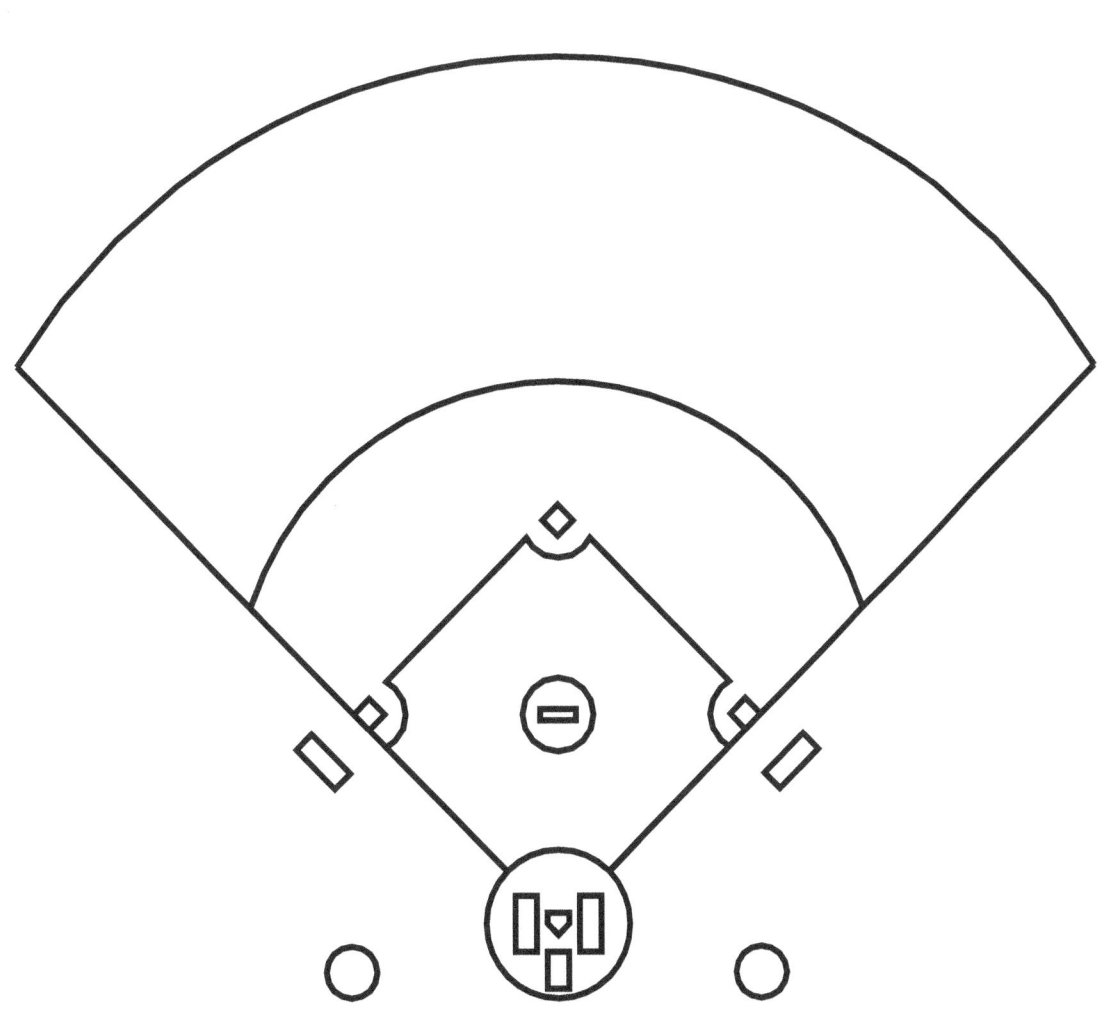

PRE-SEASON PRACTICE

Date:

Location:

My focus this week is:

Coach's focus this week is:

Skills I need to work on this week are:

I showed good sportsmanship this week by:

How I feel starting out:

This week's practice notes:

PRACTICE DAY

Date:

Location:

My focus this week is:

Coach's focus this week is:

Skills I need to work on this week are:

I showed good sportsmanship this week by:

How I feel starting out:

This week's practice notes:

GAME DAY

Date:

Opponent:

Location:

My focus today is:

Coach's focus today is:

Skills I need to work on this week are:

I showed good sportsmanship today by:

How I feel starting out:

Game Day notes:

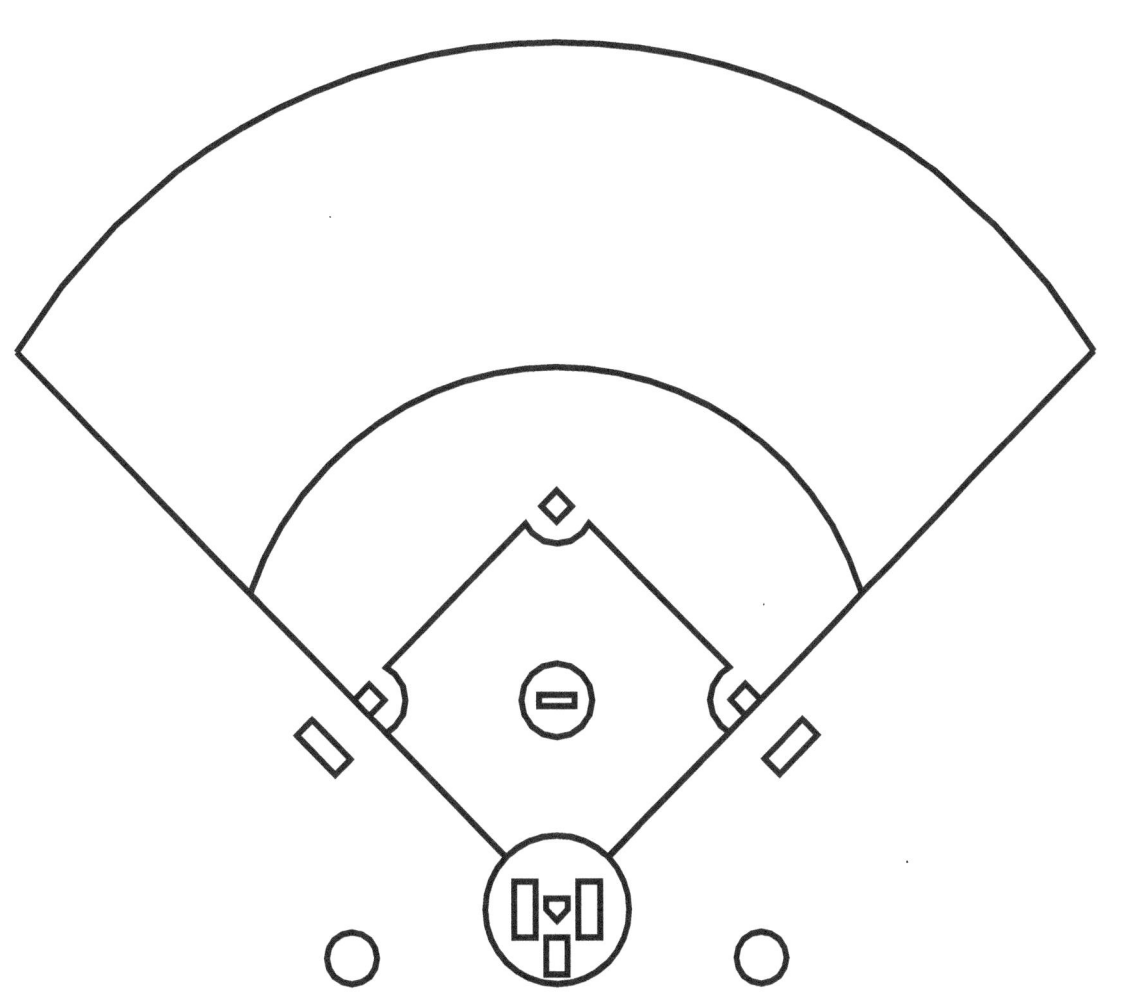

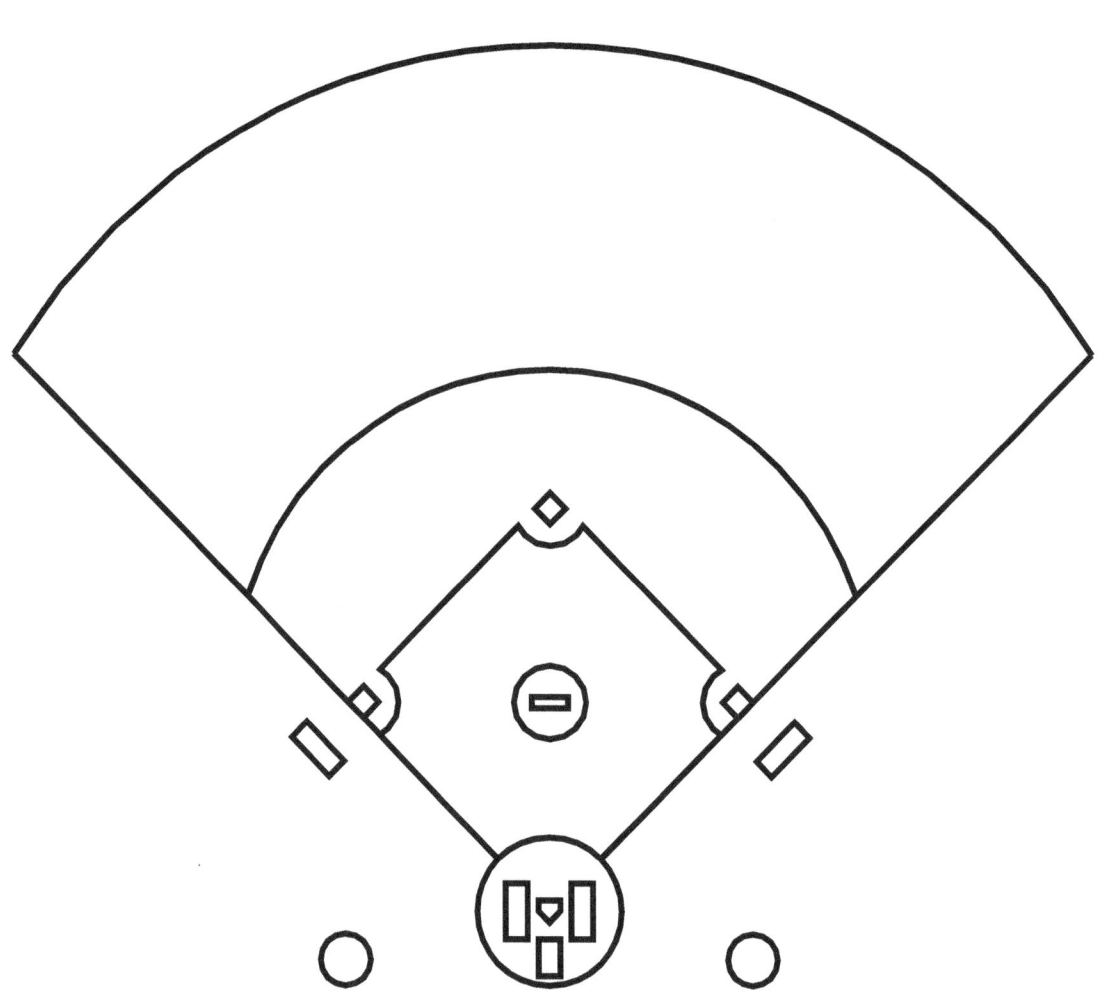

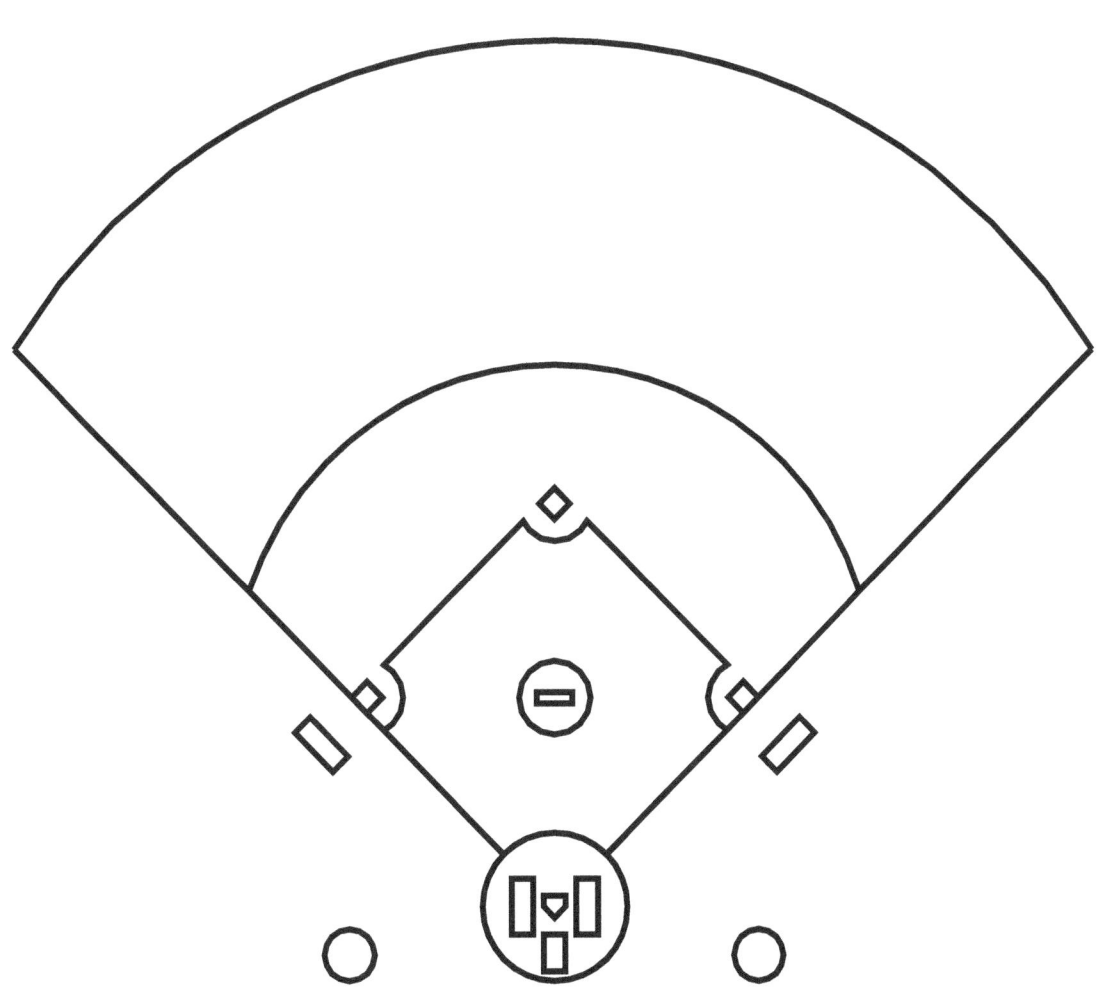

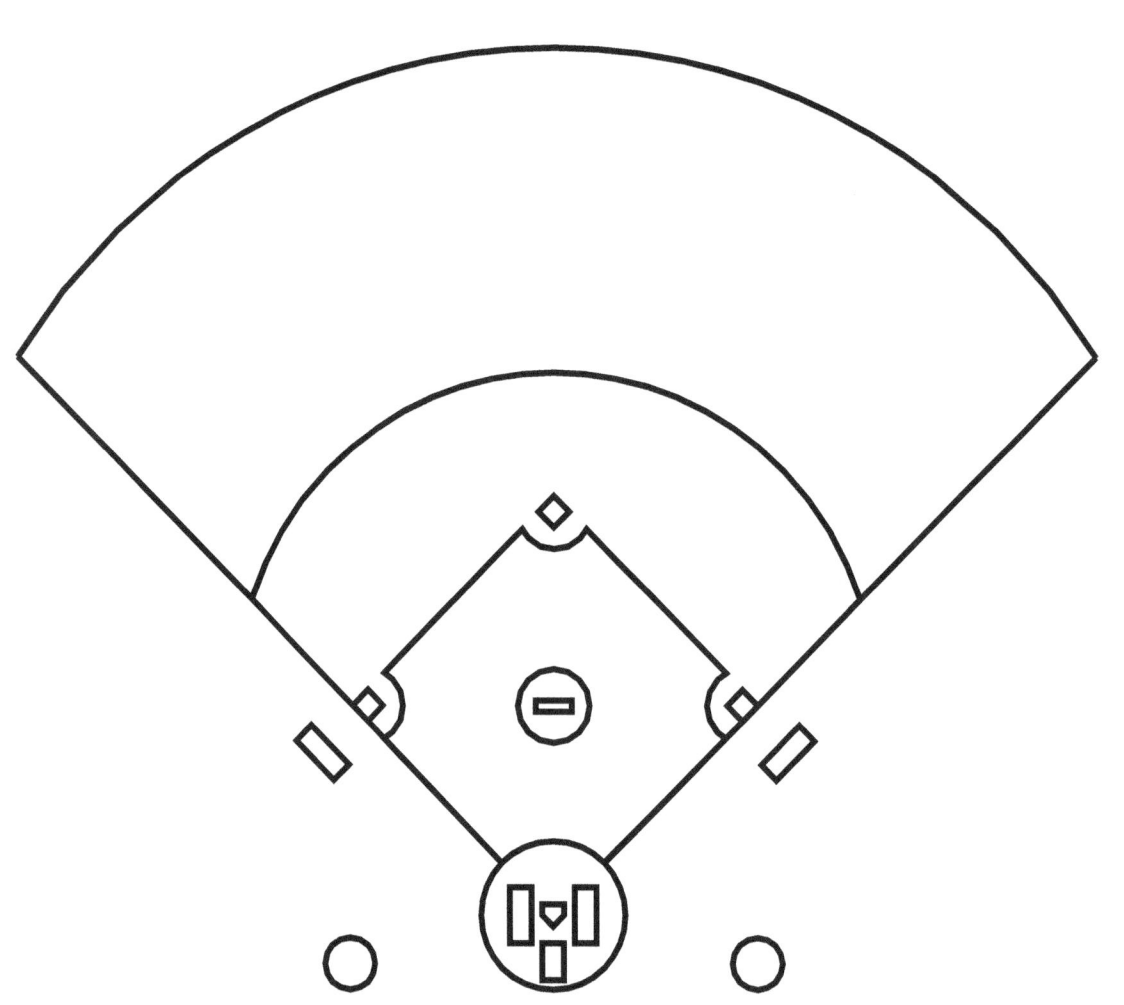

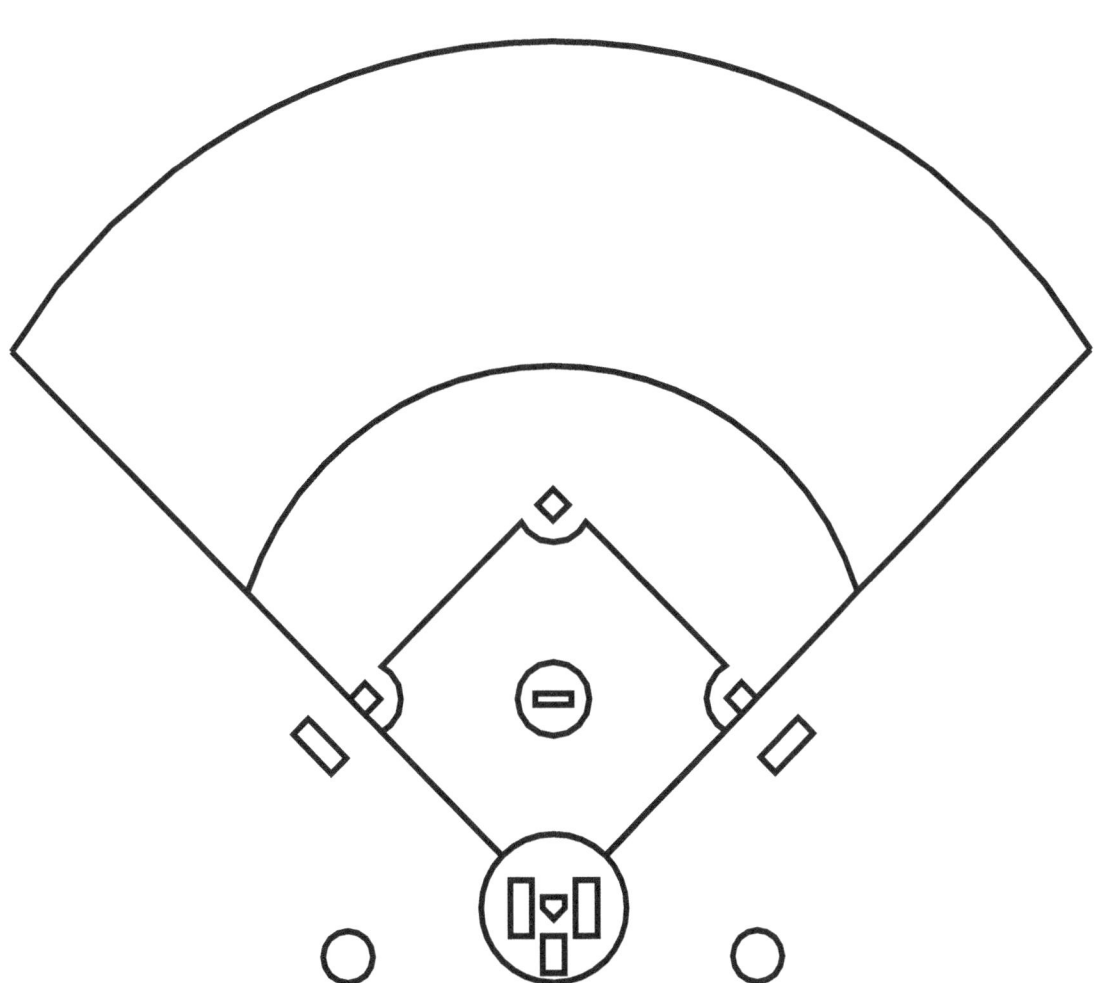

PRE-SEASON PRACTICE

Date:

Location:

My focus this week is:

Coach's focus this week is:

Skills I need to work on this week are:

I showed good sportsmanship this week by:

How I feel starting out:

This week's practice notes:

PRACTICE DAY

Date:

Location:

My focus this week is:

Coach's focus this week is:

Skills I need to work on this week are:

I showed good sportsmanship this week by:

How I feel starting out:

This week's practice notes:

GAME DAY

Date:

Opponent:

Location:

My focus today is:

Coach's focus today is:

Skills I need to work on this week are:

I showed good sportsmanship today by:

How I feel starting out:

Game Day notes:

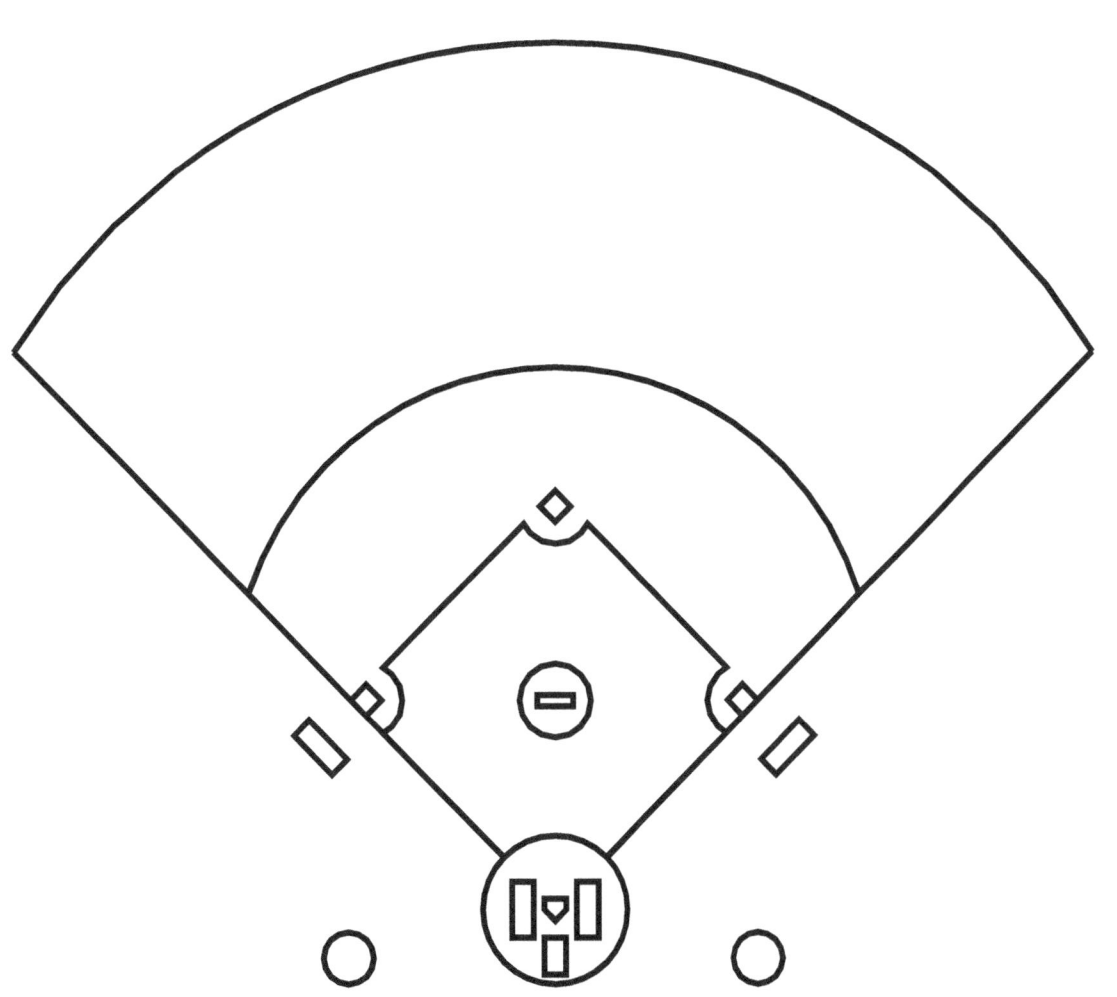

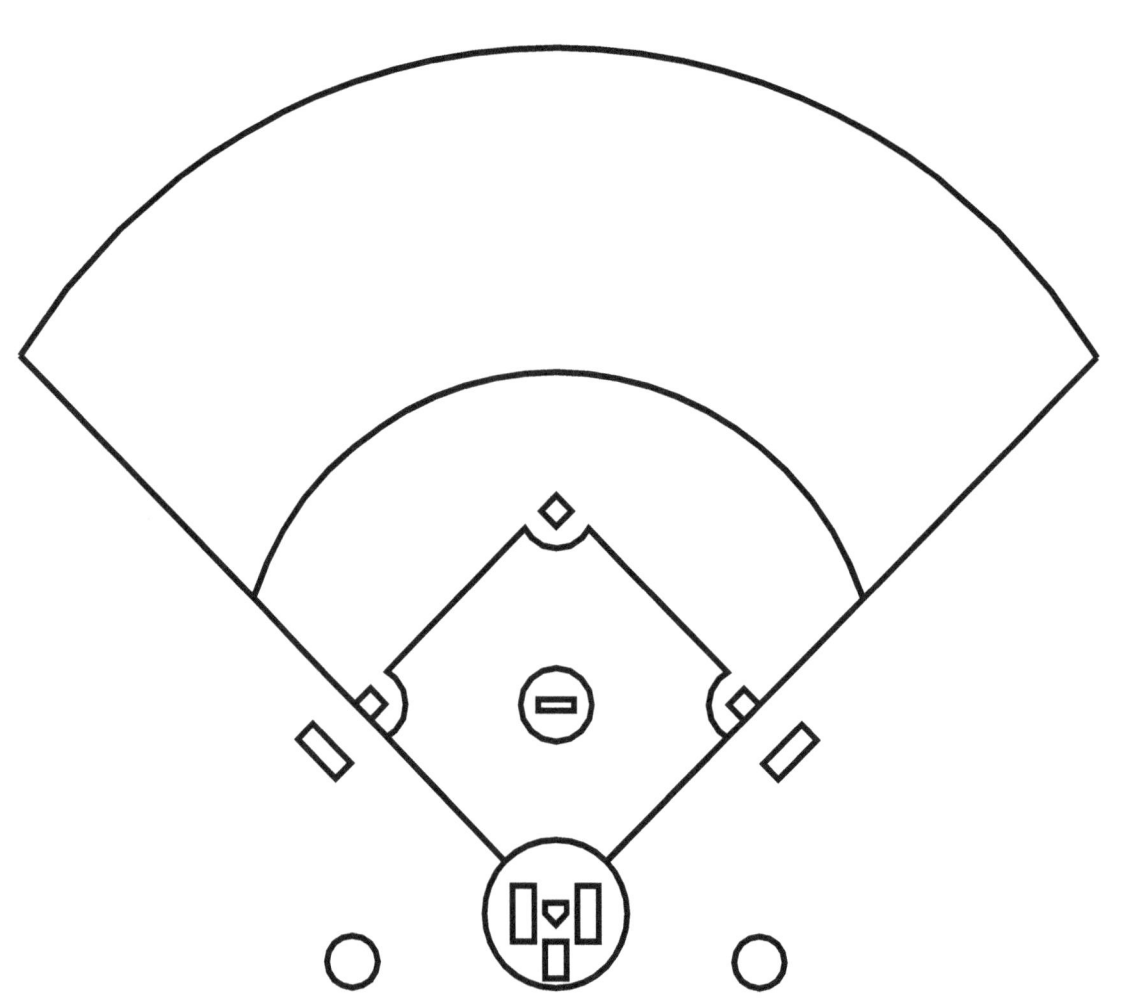

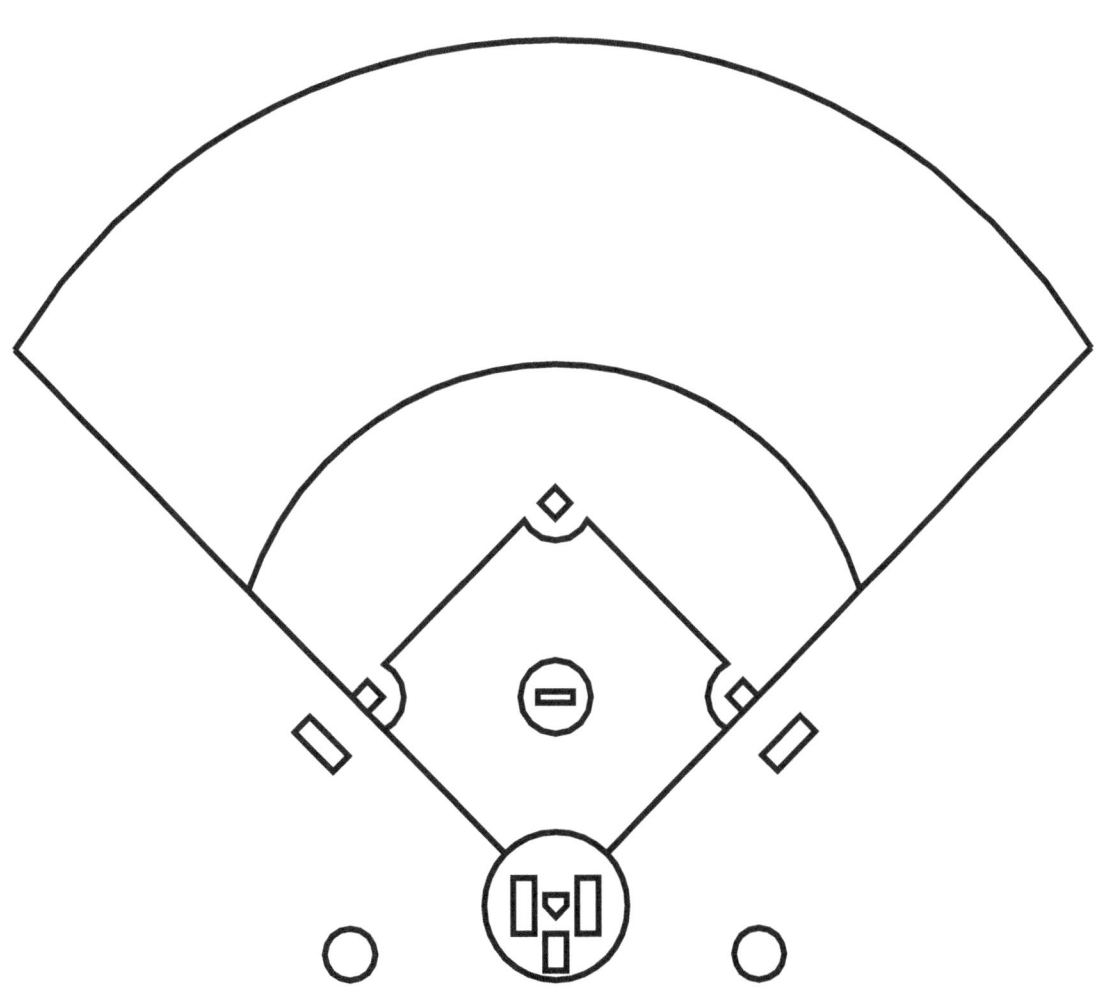

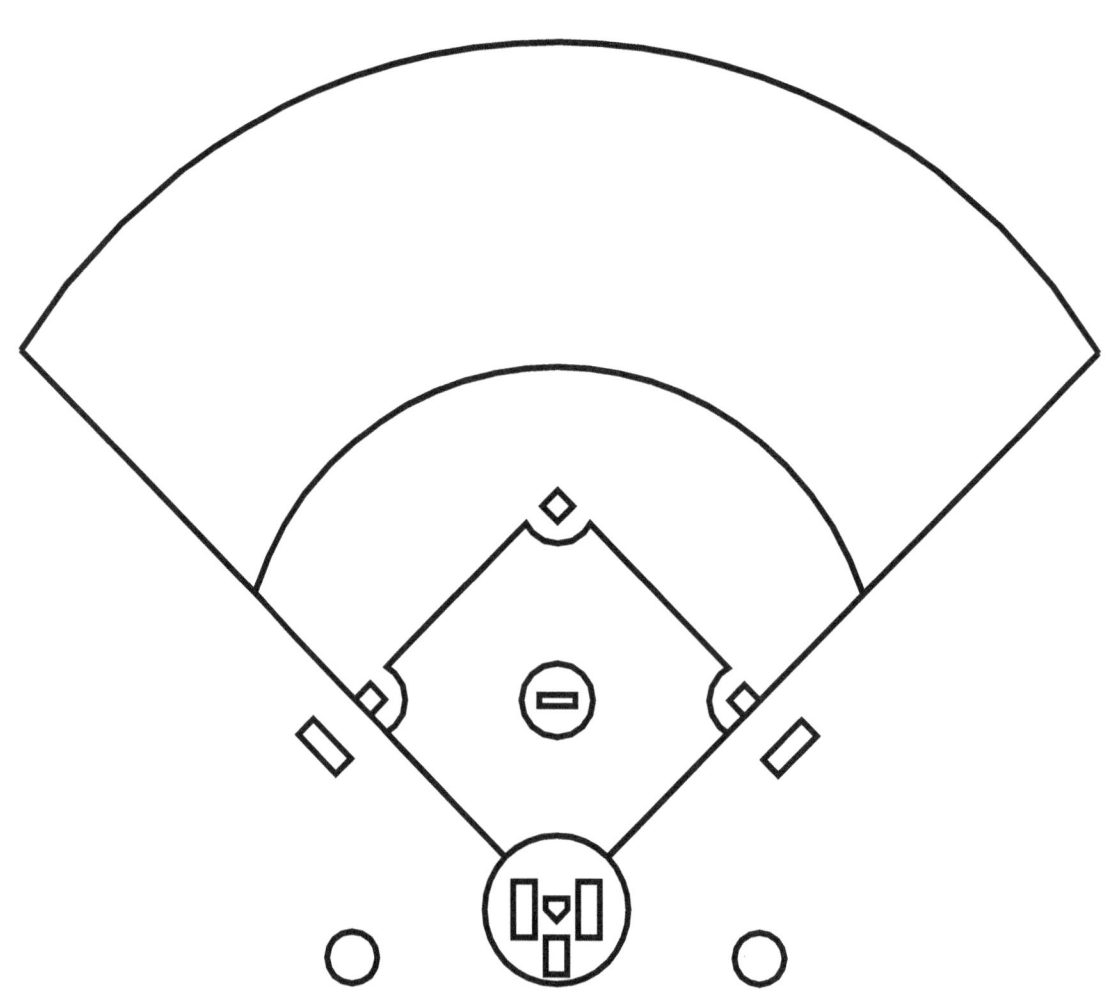

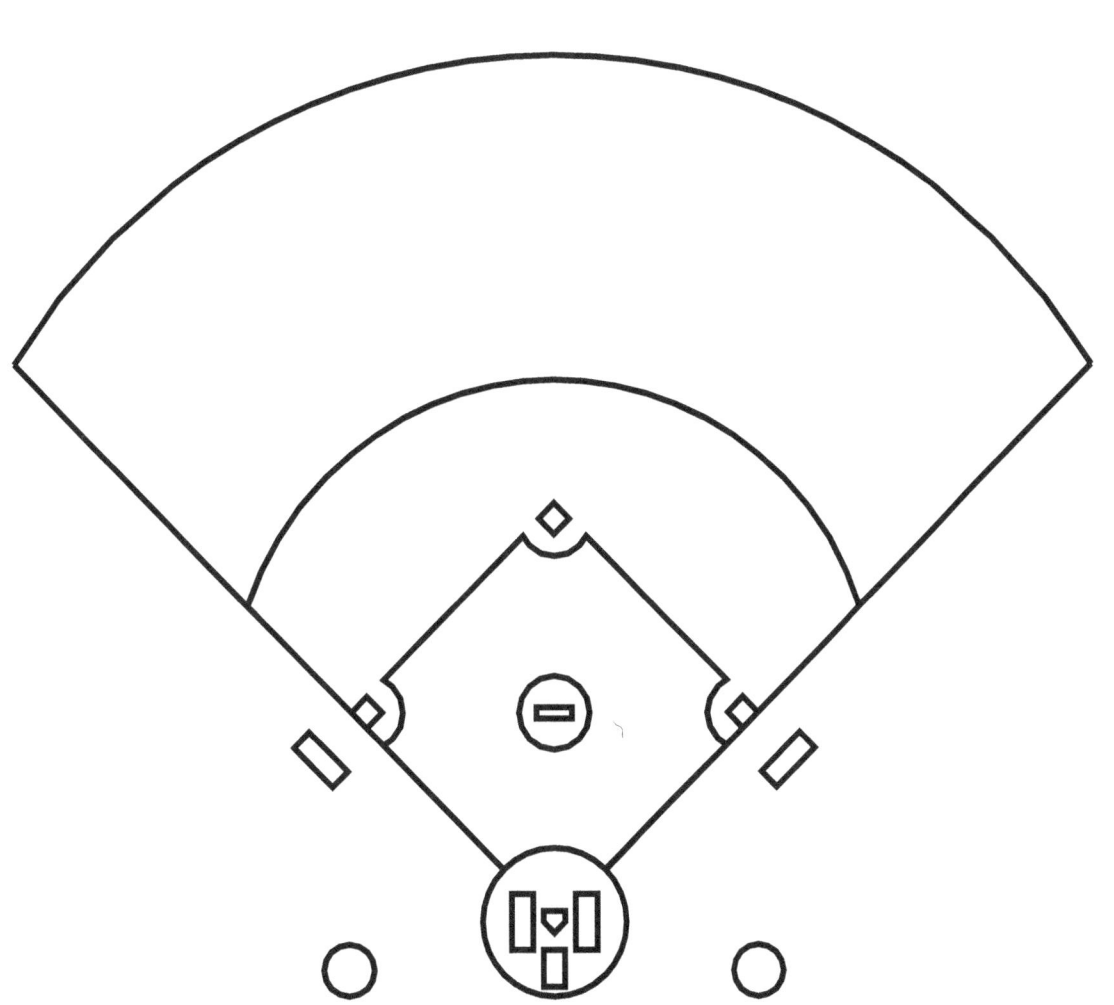

PRE-SEASON PRACTICE

Date:

Location:

My focus this week is:

Coach's focus this week is:

Skills I need to work on this week are:

I showed good sportsmanship this week by:

How I feel starting out:

This week's practice notes:

PRACTICE DAY

Date:

Location:

My focus this week is:

Coach's focus this week is:

Skills I need to work on this week are:

I showed good sportsmanship this week by:

How I feel starting out:

This week's practice notes:

GAME DAY

Date:

Opponent:

Location:

My focus today is:

Coach's focus today is:

Skills I need to work on this week are:

I showed good sportsmanship today by:

How I feel starting out:

Game Day notes:

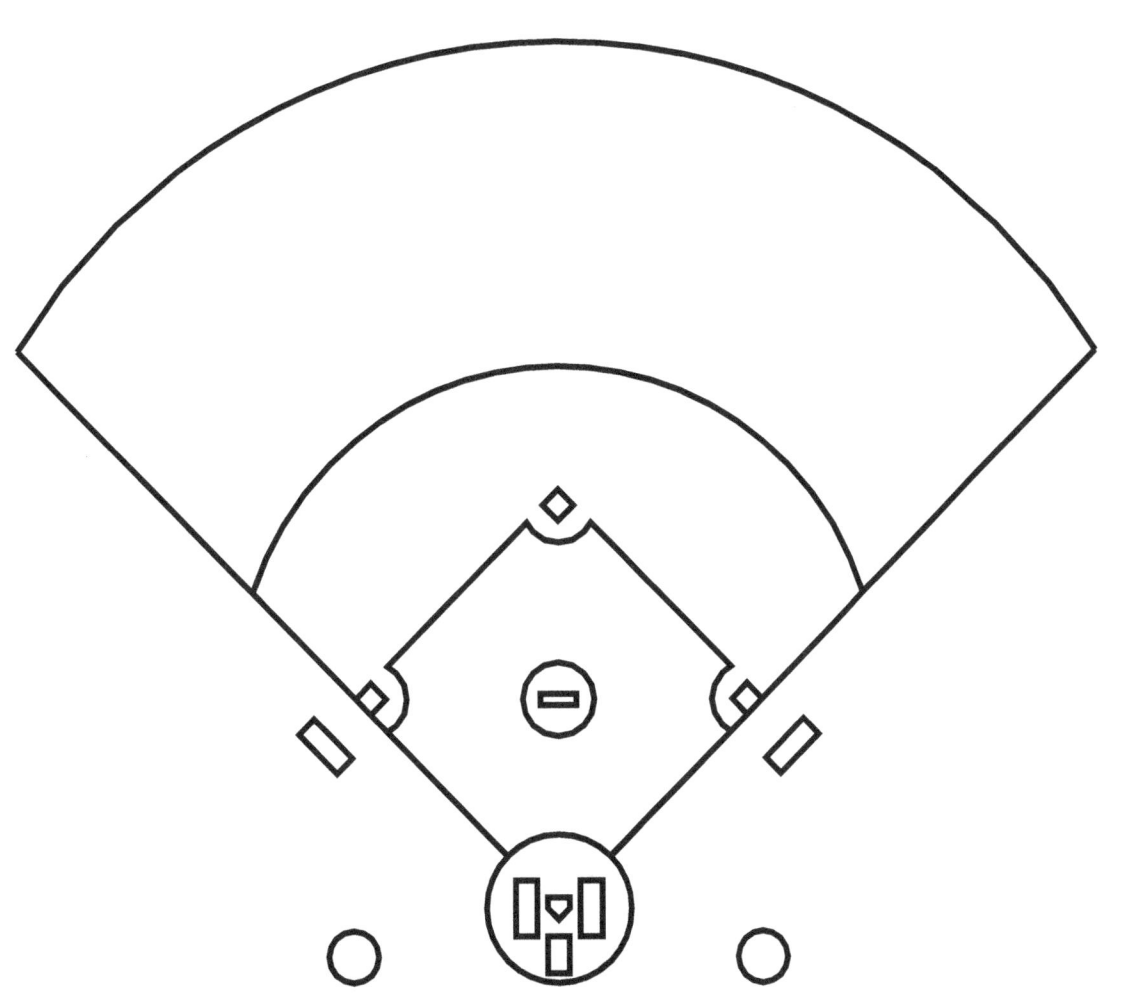

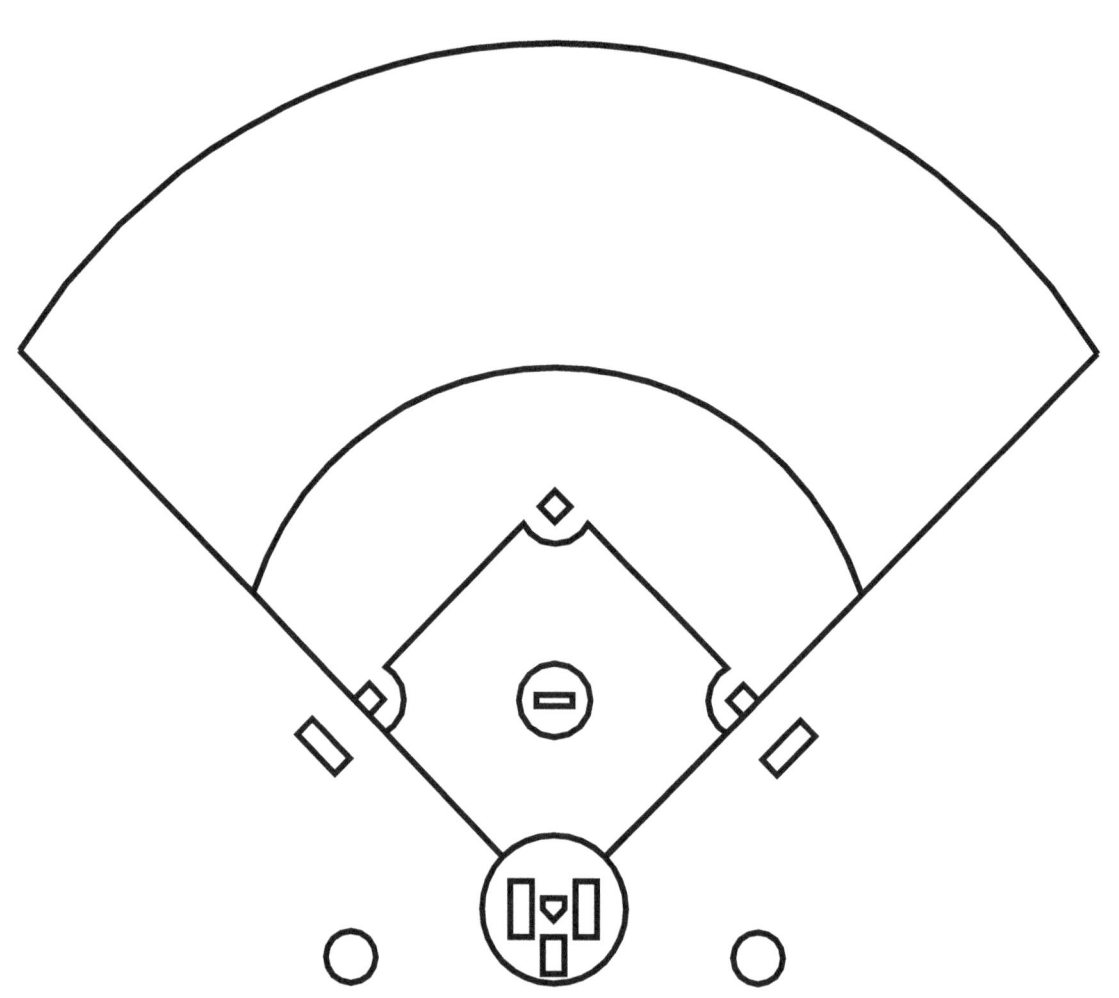

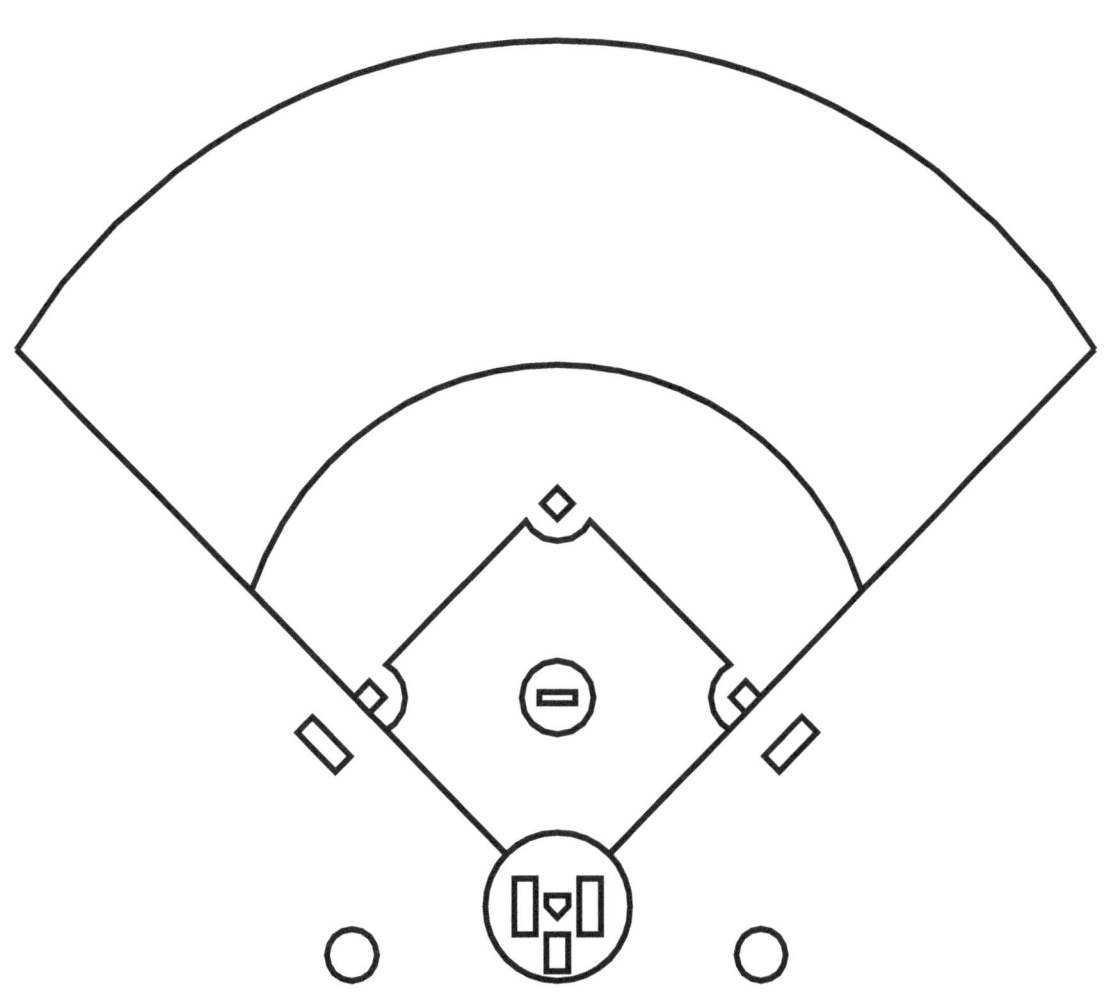

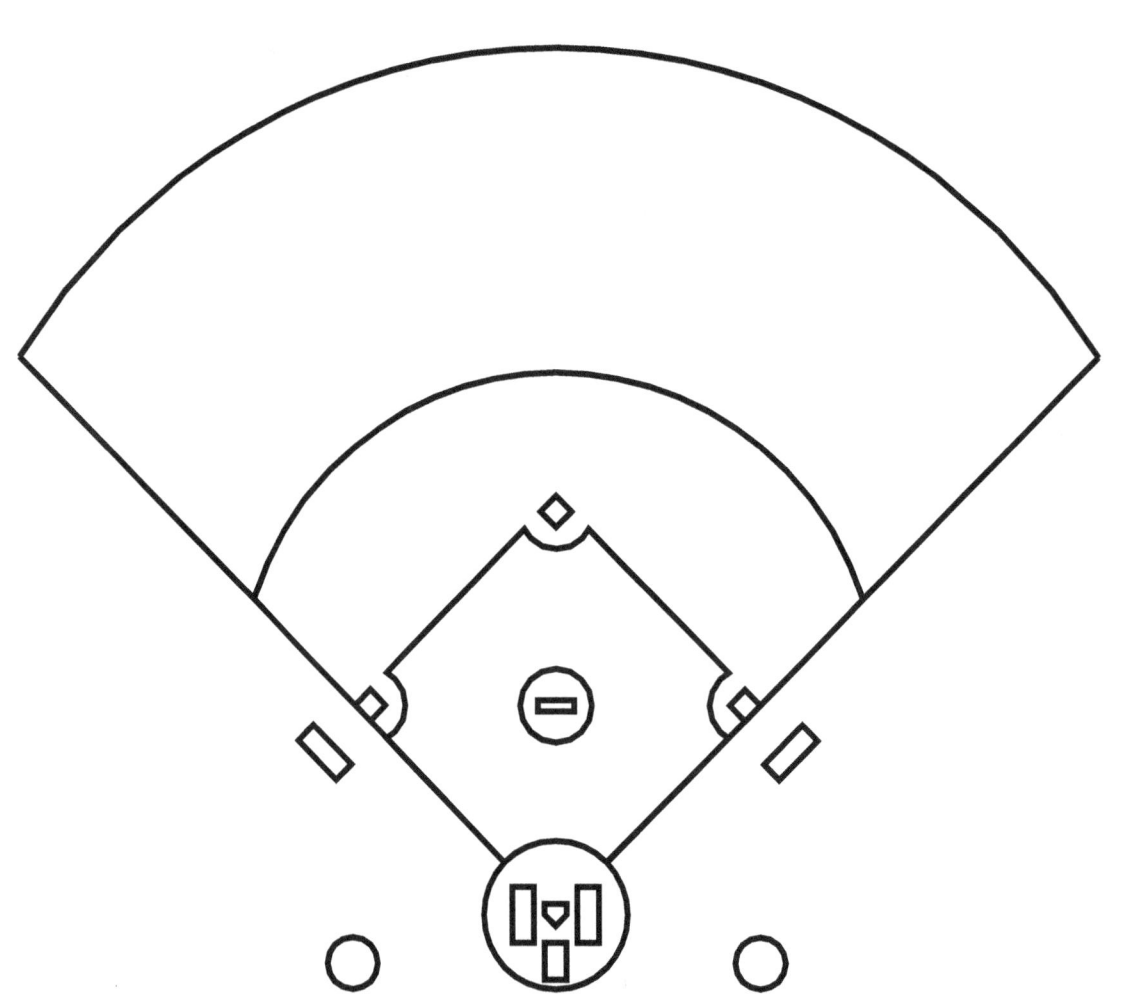

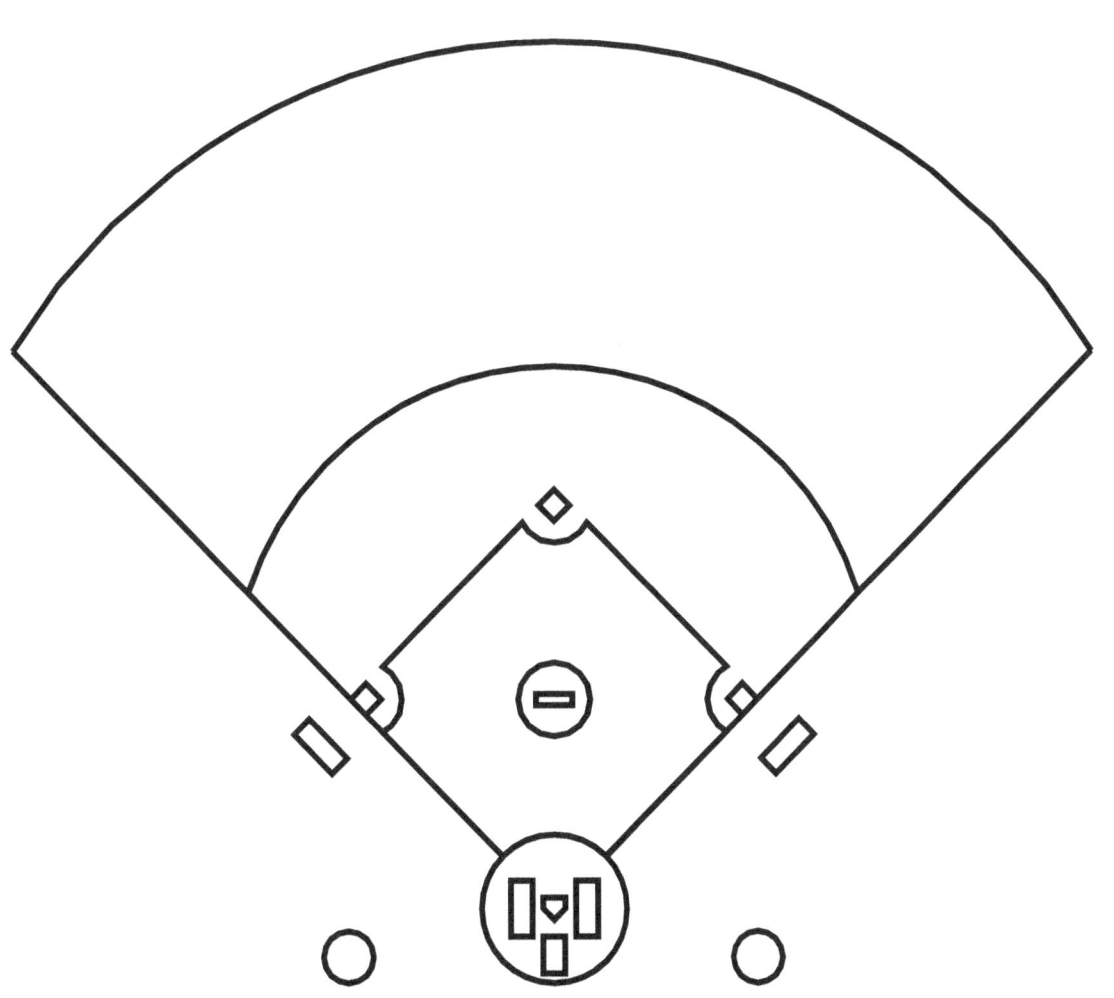

PRE-SEASON PRACTICE

Date:

Location:

My focus this week is:

Coach's focus this week is:

Skills I need to work on this week are:

I showed good sportsmanship this week by:

How I feel starting out:

This week's practice notes:

PRACTICE DAY

Date:

Location:

My focus this week is:

Coach's focus this week is:

Skills I need to work on this week are:

I showed good sportsmanship this week by:

How I feel starting out:

This week's practice notes:

GAME DAY

Date:

Opponent:

Location:

My focus today is:

Coach's focus today is:

Skills I need to work on this week are:

I showed good sportsmanship today by:

How I feel starting out:

Game Day notes:

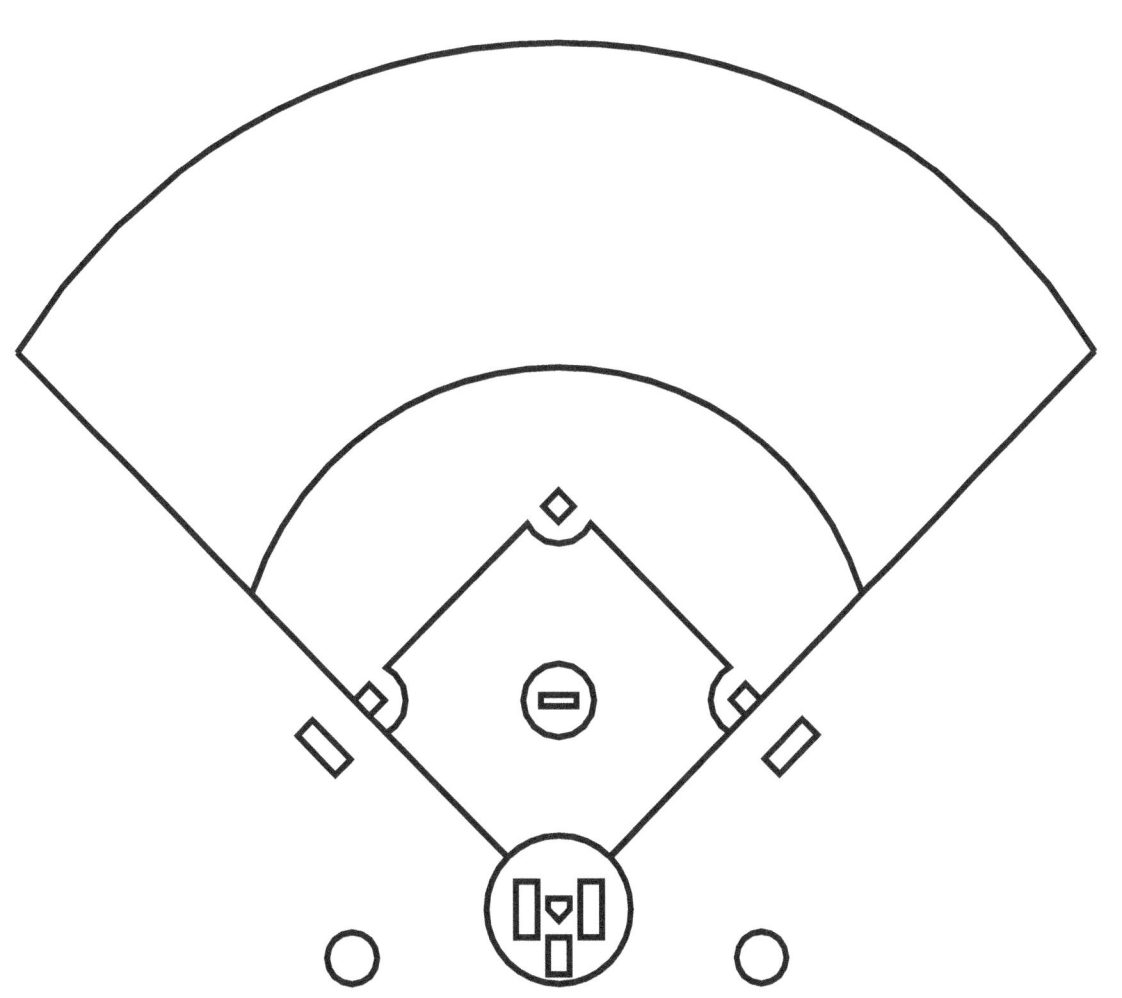

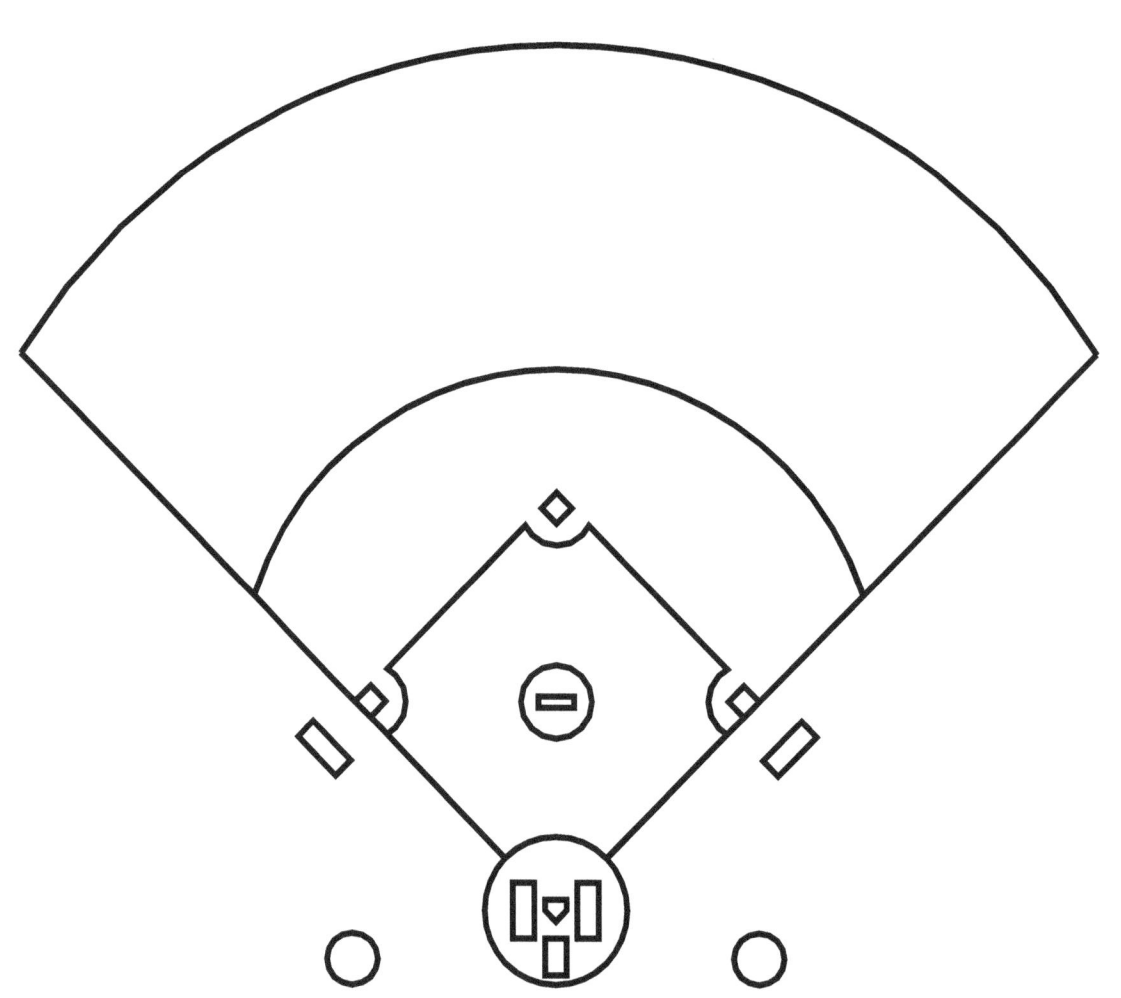

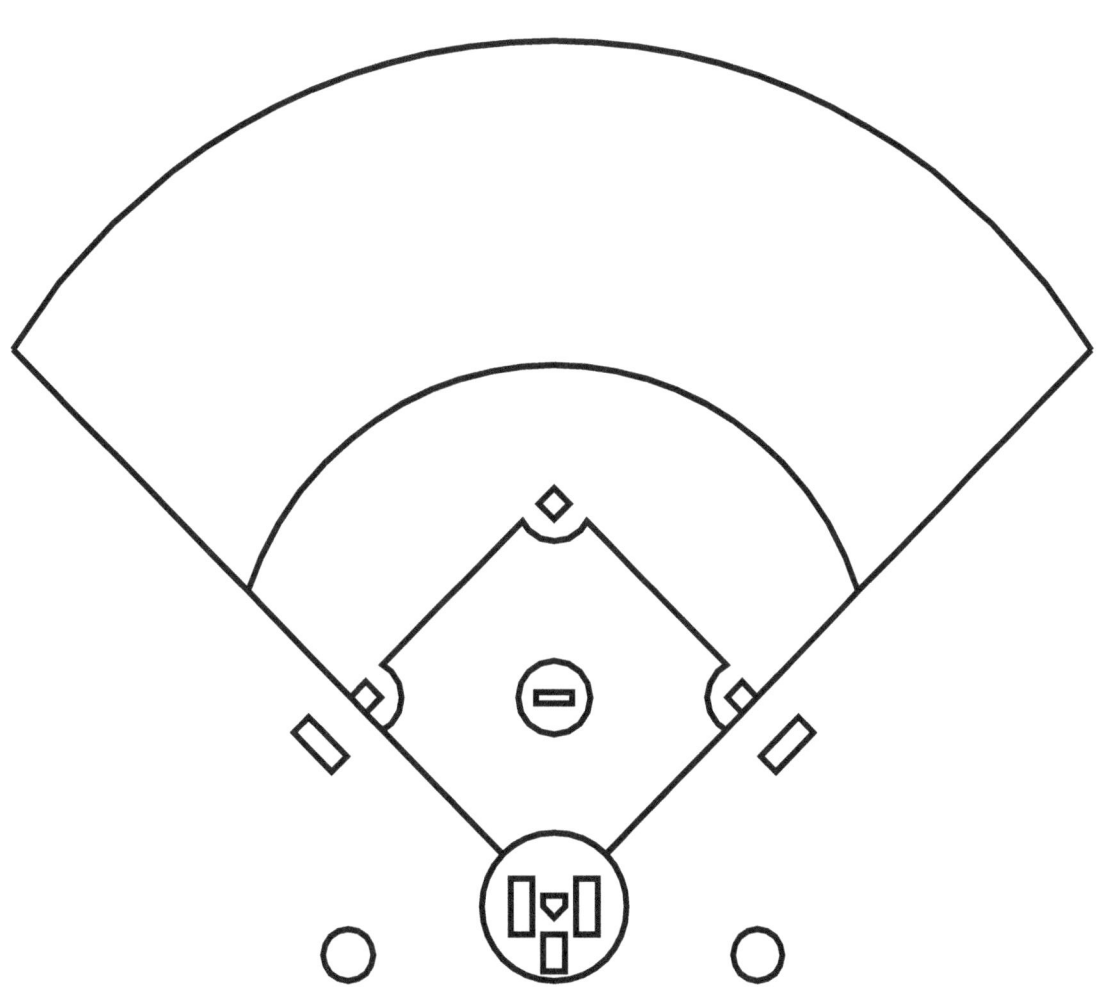

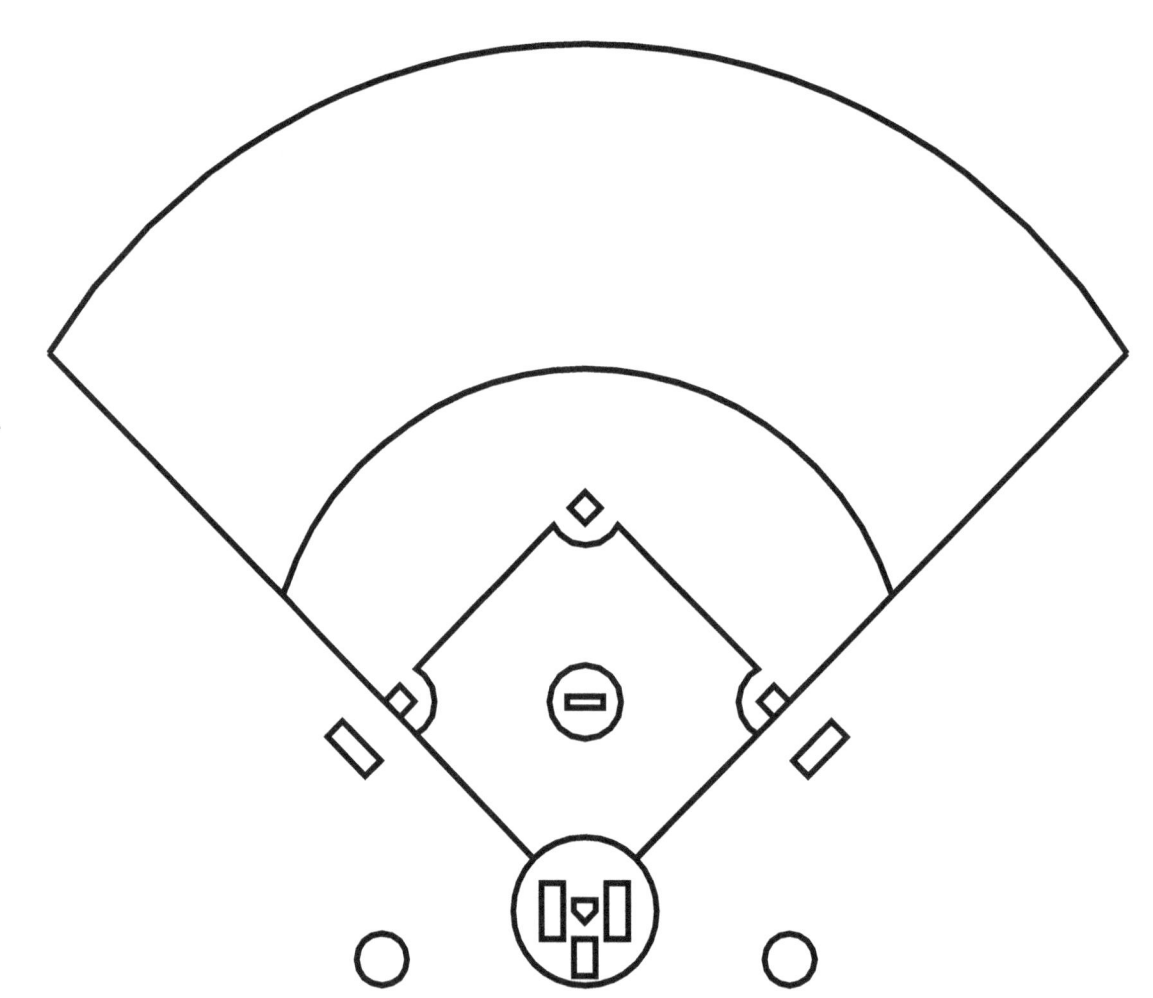

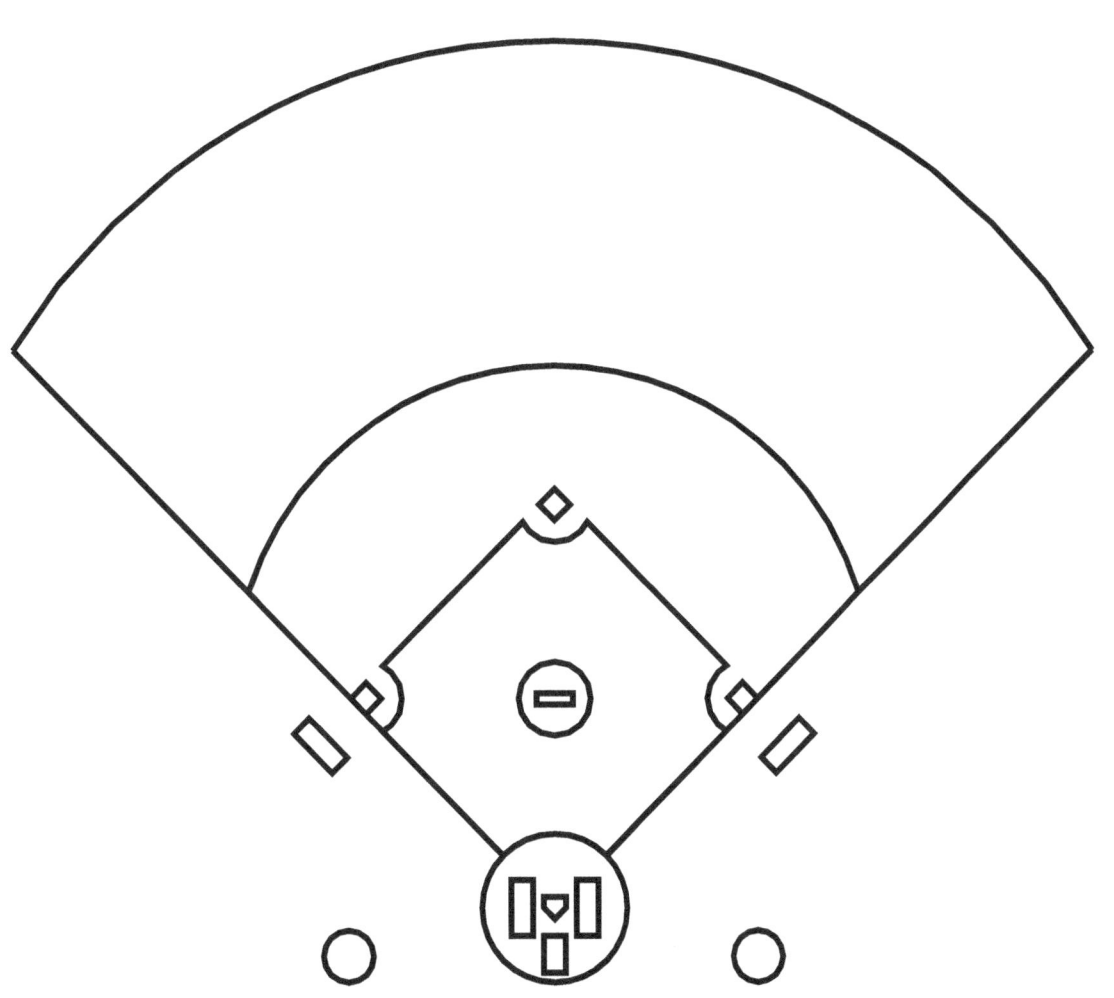

PRE-SEASON PRACTICE

Date:

Location:

My focus this week is:

Coach's focus this week is:

Skills I need to work on this week are:

I showed good sportsmanship this week by:

How I feel starting out:

This week's practice notes:

PRACTICE DAY

Date:

Location:

My focus this week is:

Coach's focus this week is:

Skills I need to work on this week are:

I showed good sportsmanship this week by:

How I feel starting out:

This week's practice notes:

GAME DAY

Date:

Opponent:

Location:

My focus today is:

Coach's focus today is:

Skills I need to work on this week are:

I showed good sportsmanship today by:

How I feel starting out:

Game Day notes:

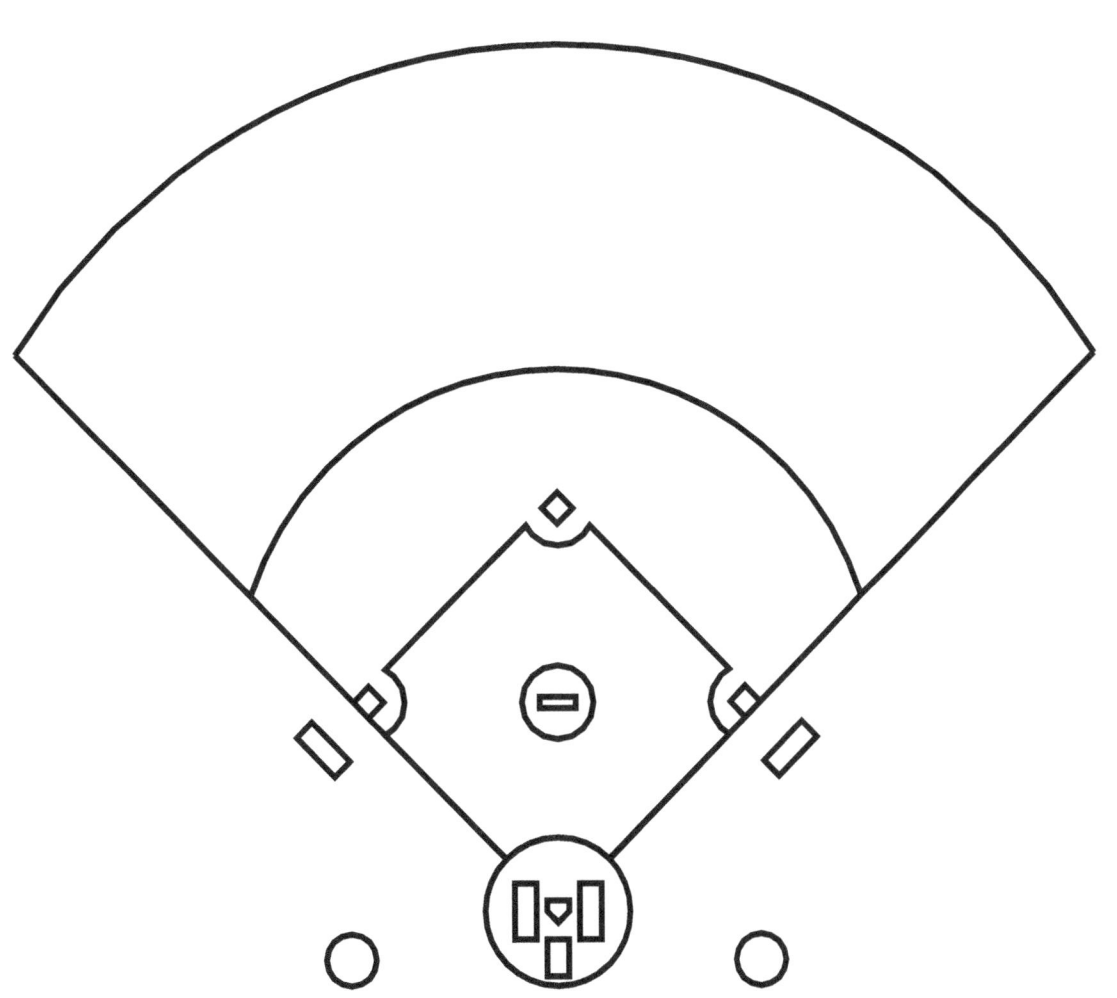

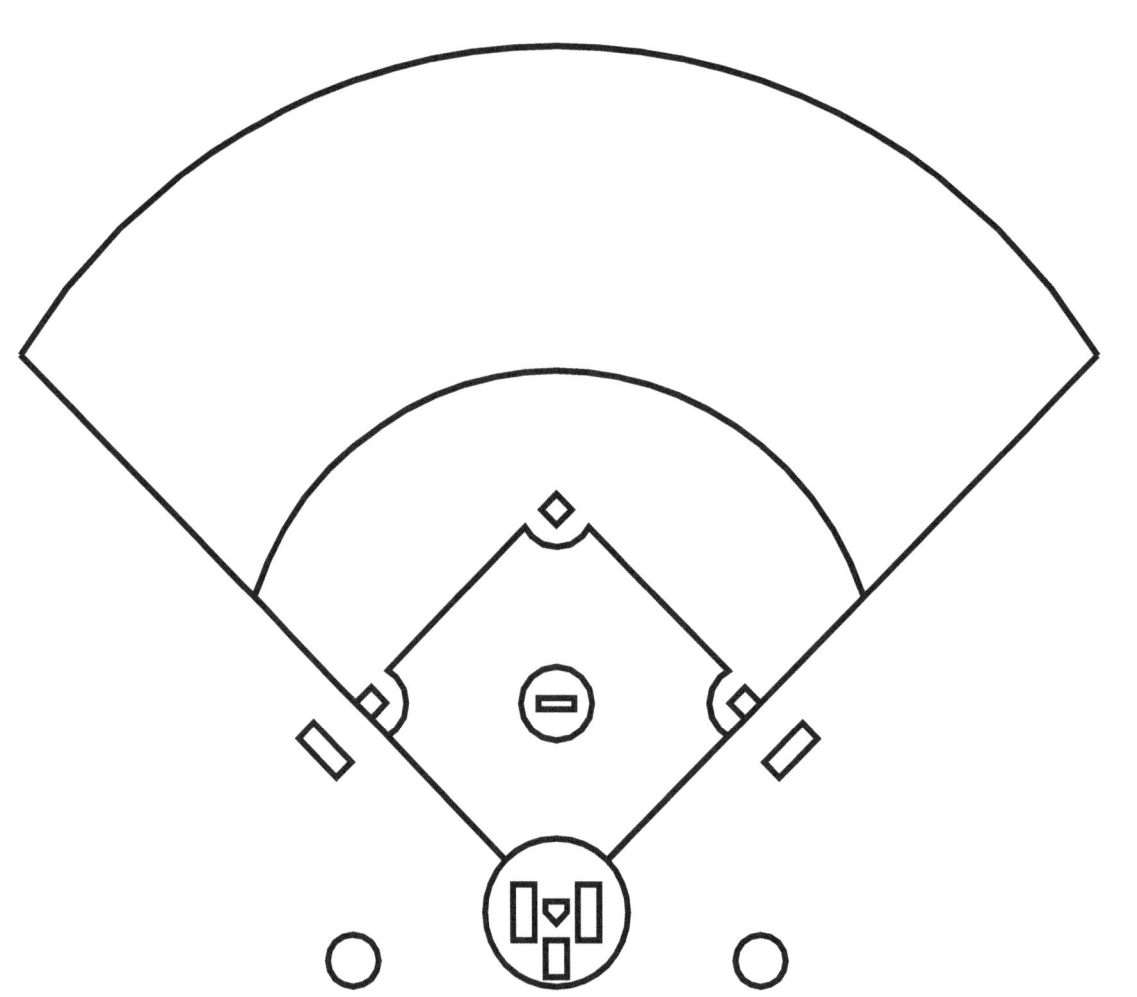

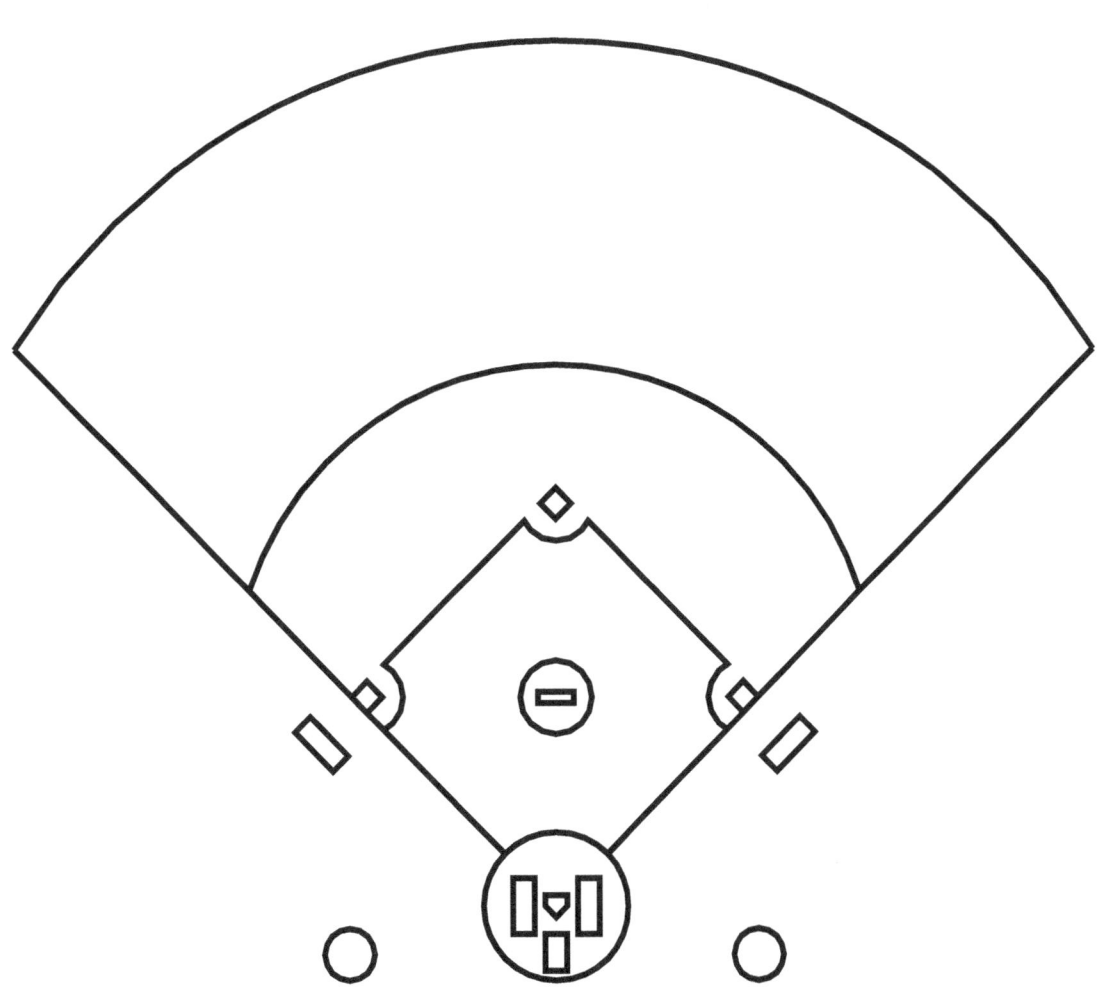

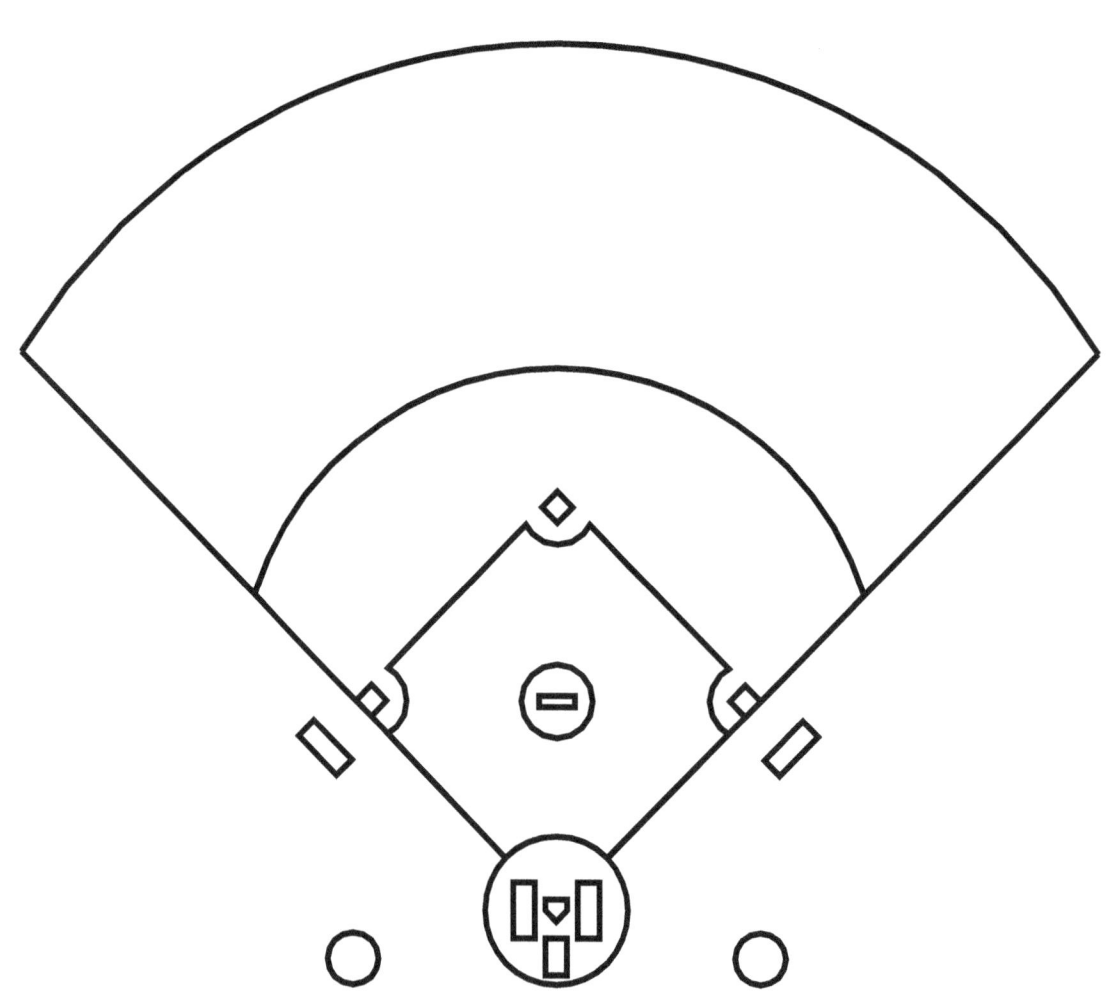

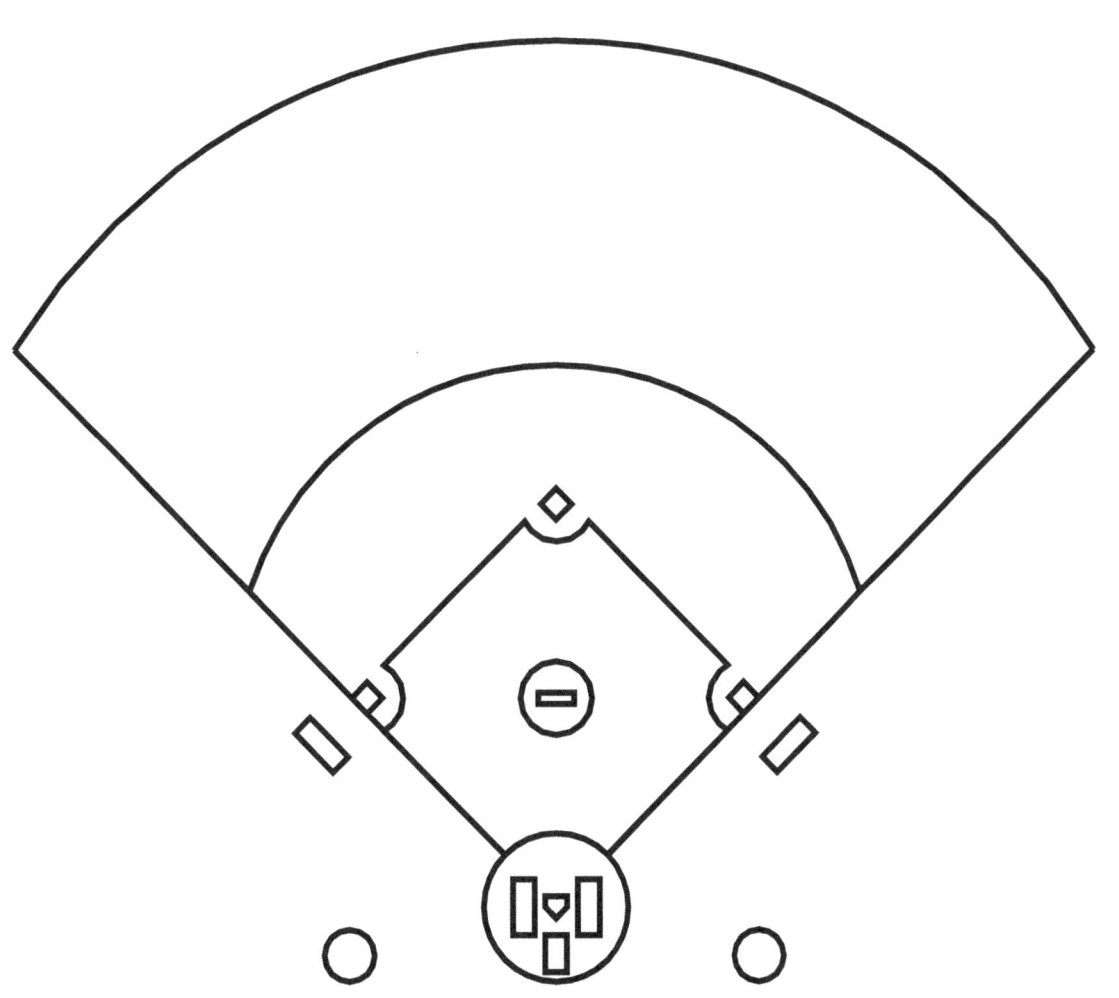

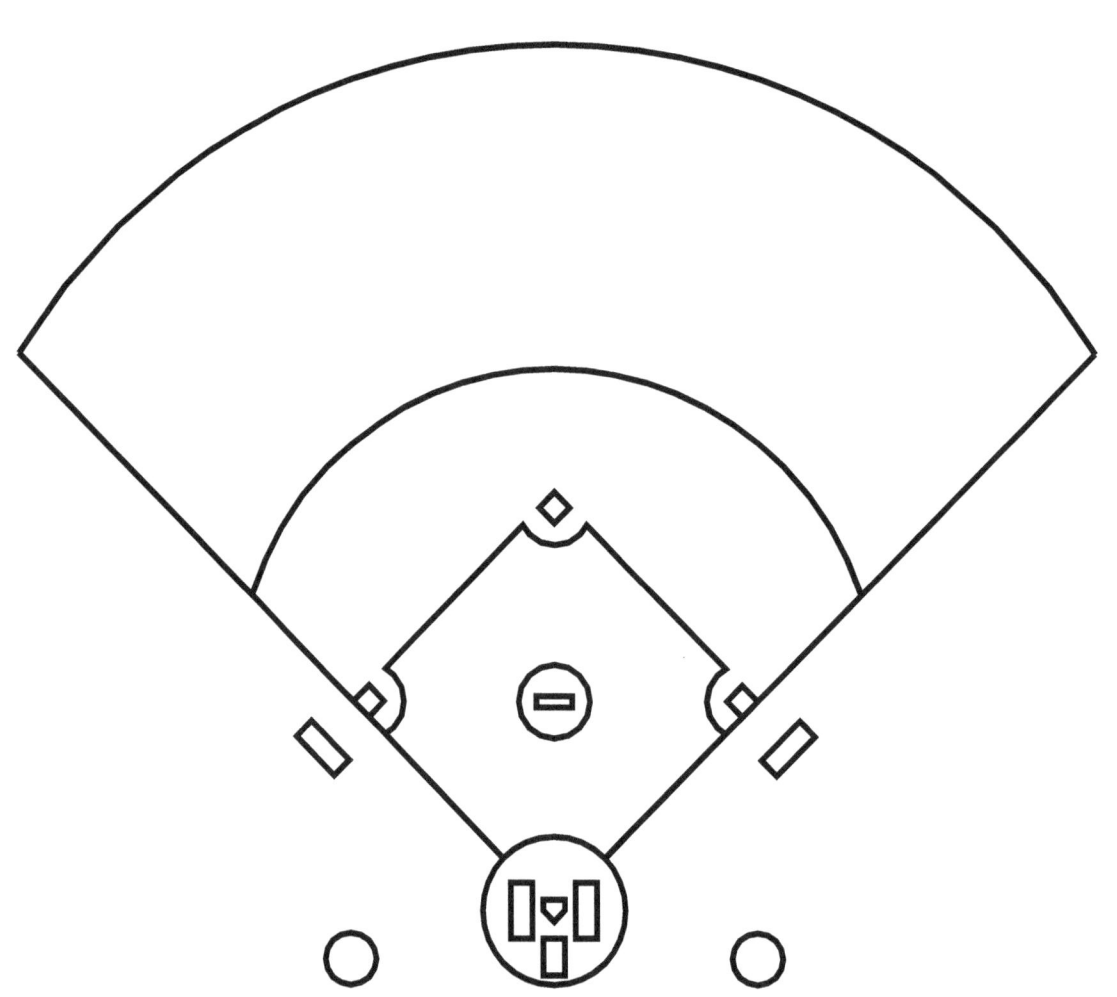

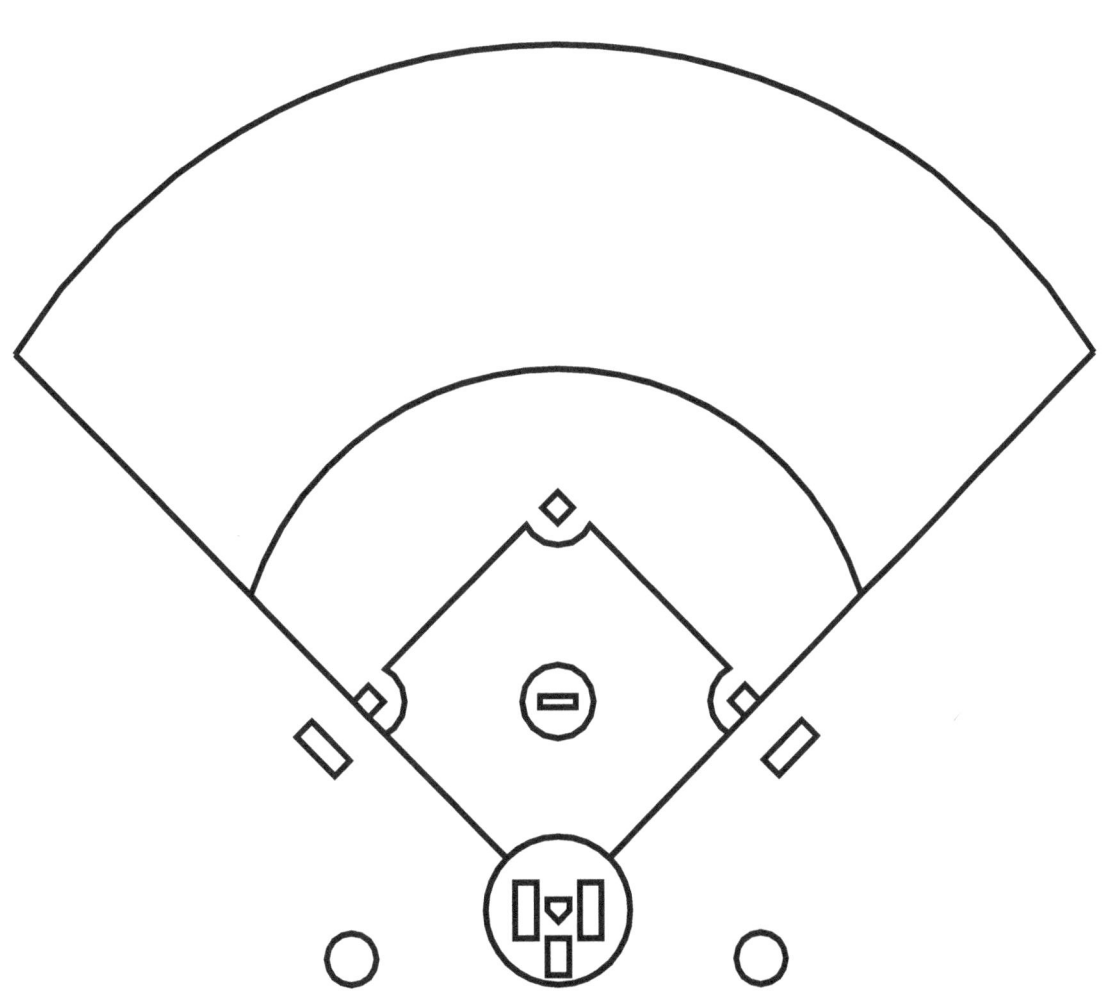

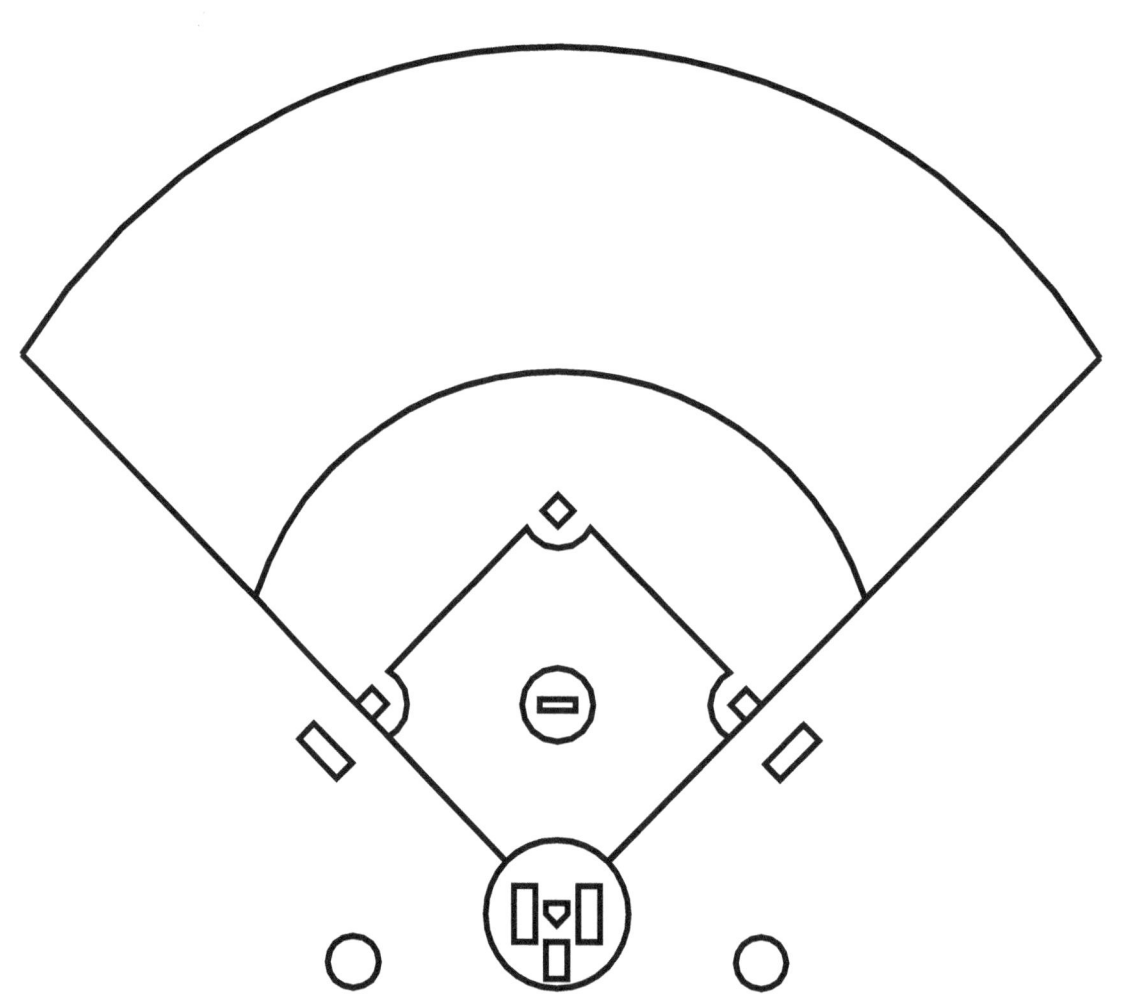

www.ingramcontent.com/pod-product-compliance
Lightning Source LLC
Chambersburg PA
CBHW082207090526
44583CB00021BA/2856